A GUIDE TO BUILDING FITNESS TRAILS

JUDY GILL, Ph.D.

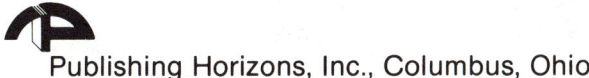
Publishing Horizons, Inc., Columbus, Ohio

GV
462
.G55
1986

©Copyright 1986, PUBLISHING HORIZONS, INC.
2950 North High Street
P.O. Box 02190
Columbus, Ohio 43202

ALL RIGHTS RESERVED. No part of this publication may be reproduced, stored in a retrieval system, or transmitted, in any form or by any means, electronic, mechanical, photocopying, recording or otherwise, without prior written permission of the copyright holder.

Printed in the United States.

1   2   3   4   7   6   5   4

Library of Congress Cataloging in Publication Data

Gill, Judy.
   A guide to building fitness trails.

   Originally published: Parcours. Pierrefonds, Que. : Palmquist Publications, c1977.
     Bibliography: p.
     Includes index.
     1. Circuit training. 2. Physical fitness.
3. Circuit training--Design and construction. I. Title.
GV462.G55   1986   712'.5   85-30106
ISBN 0-942280-21-0

Photographs By

Barry McGee

Artwork By

John Starkey

CONTENTS

1. WHY A FITNESS TRAIL? 1
2. A WORD ABOUT GENERAL FITNESS 6
3. PULSE RATE-BASED FITNESS PROGRAMS 23
4. HOW TO SET UP A FITNESS PROGRAM 29
5. STEPS IN CONSTRUCTING A FITNESS TRAIL 31
   BIBLIOGRAPHY 74

WHY A FITNESS TRAIL?

Millions of dollars have been spent making North Americans aware of their lack of physical fitness. But once aware, then what?

Some valuable lessons can be learned from our European counterparts. Fitness is a family affair in Europe, a daily part of the people's lives. Mass participation is emphasized rather than elite sport. One of their innovative programs, the fitness trail, was developed to suit these needs.

The fitness trail is a jogging circuit located in the outdoors. Exercise stations are located along a pathway. You run from station to station, stop, do the exercise indicated, and proceed to the next one. Thus, you combine both a cardiovascular and muscular workout into one.

The fitness trail is an idea that originated in Switzerland with the Vita Life Insurance Company during the 1960s. Concerned about the poor physical condition of the Swiss people, Vita inaugurated the first trail in a park in Zurich. The response surpassed their wildest dreams. Today, fitness trails can be found throughout Europe and the Scandinavian countries.

The beauty of a fitness trail is that you can exercise while enjoying the surrounding scenery. What to some is unpleasant calisthenics becomes more appealing through the addition of scenic woodlands and fresh air.

People need a place to go which is inexpensive and where they can be assured of a good fitness program; which is readily accessible; a place where friends and family can exercise in the outdoors in pleasant surroundings with no one to compete with but themselves. A fitness trail is the answer.

Then why not simply import the European version? Its main drawback is that it is open for the summer season only. We have also learned over the years that some of their exercises can be dangerous. What we need is a fitness trail of North American orientation, one that is suited to our unique climatic conditions, a trail that is open 24 hours a day, 365 days a year. Fitness is not a "summer only" pursuit.

There is no reason why every community in North America cannot have at least one fitness trail. Properly designed and equipped trails can cost less than $5,000 to erect. For this small amount, North Americans can be assured of obtaining a safe, practical, and well-balanced conditioning program.

With the above in mind, this book came into being—to offer guidelines in constructing an inexpensive and safe fitness trail, suited for North American needs.

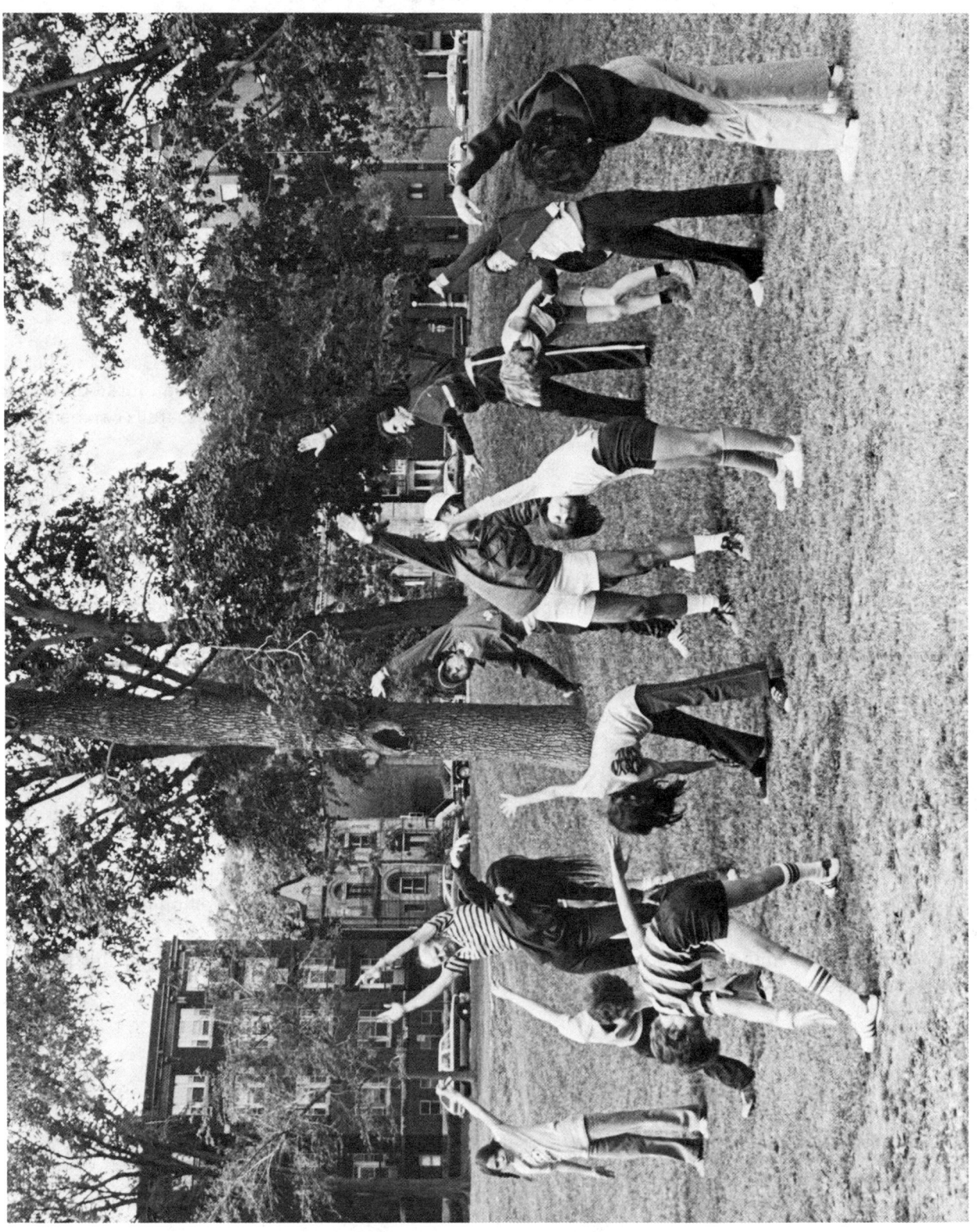

FITNESS TRAIL OBJECTIVES

The general aim of any fitness trail is to promote fitness. Specifically, it is to create a trail which:

1. Will incorporate all basic fitness principles.

2. Provides a safe and enjoyable conditioning program.

3. Develops both cardiovascular and muscular fitness.

4. Includes a warm-up and cool-down as part of the program.

5. Can be used all year long (all exercises can be done on foot in summer; on cross-country skis in the winter).

6. Is open 24 hours a day.

7. Is free of charge.

8. Promotes family and individual fitness.

9. Can be used by a large number of people simultaneously.

10. Enables people of varying heights, ages, and sexes to participate together.

11. Is adaptable to varying levels of physical condition from very poor to excellent.

12. Can be used as a training course for people with different interests in sport: professional, amateur, or recreational.

13. Is outdoors.

14. Is bilingual (if necessary).

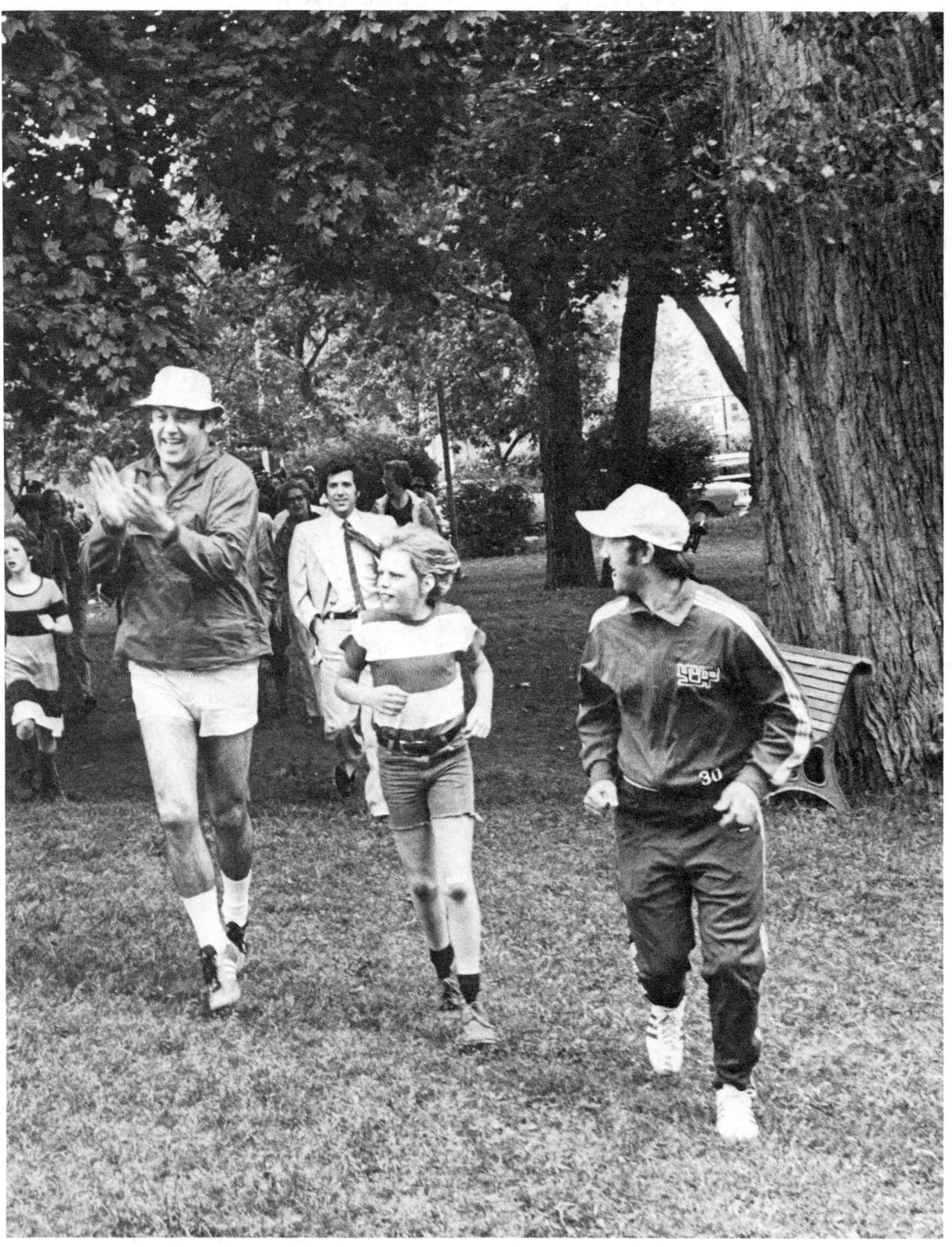

WHO CAN USE THE FITNESS TRAIL?

EVERYONE!!!

It is available without supervision 24 hours a day all year long, with no cost to the participants themselves. No incredible skill is required and you don't compete against anyone except yourself.

It can be used simultaneously by a large number of people of differing body builds and ages. It provides for varying levels of physical conditioning from very poor to excellent and it can be used as a training course for people with a variety of interests in sport, professional, amateur, or recreational.

The short circuit enables young children and senior citizens to take part. Advanced-level participants who wish to run a longer distance than that of the trail can try this plan. Run the fitness trail twice. The first time do all the odd-numbered exercises and the next time all the even-numbered ones. This way you go through all the exercises but will have a longer run between stations.

Coaches! Use it as a warm-up for your practices.

Do-it-yourselfers! Use it as a pre-season conditioner for skiing, tennis, football, etc. or just for general fitness.

School children! Develop it into an enjoyable addition to the physical education program.

Families! Make it an outing for the entire family. Make fitness a family affair.

Business people! Work out at lunch or after a rough day at the office.

Weight watchers! Combine exercise with your diet program to tone up those muscles as you lose weight.

Senior citizens! There's no reason why you can't participate. Fitness is for everyone. It's never too late to start. Just proceed at a reduced pace under supervision.

North Americans need the exercise. Yet staying fit and trim need not cost a fortune. Build a fitness trail in your neighborhood.

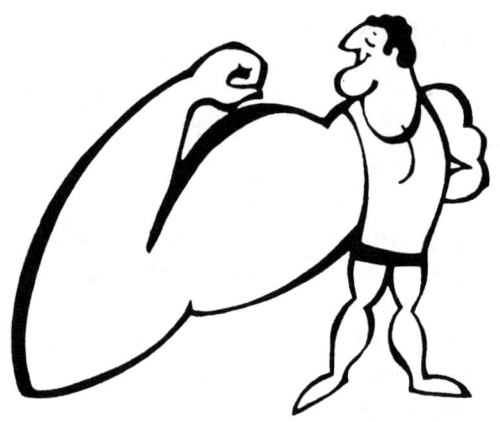 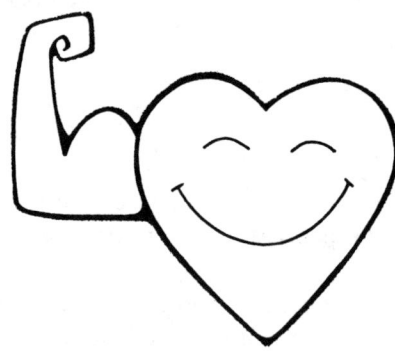

A WORD ABOUT GENERAL FITNESS

A beautiful body does not necessarily guarantee physical fitness—nor does a muscular one. There are two types of fitness—muscular and cardiovascular.

Muscular exercise is just what it says: activities that tone up muscles, eliminate flab, help you lose inches, and increase muscular strength, endurance, and flexibility. You might think of it as "external" fitness, as toned and lean muscles are readily visible. Familiar activities such as yoga, calisthenics, and weight training generally fall into this category.

"Stamina," "wind," "aerobics," or "cardiovascular" fitness all refer to exercise for the heart, lungs, and circulatory systems. Think of it as "internal" fitness including rhythmic and repetitious activities such as running, walking, rope skipping, cycling, swimming, and dance, to name just a few.

Cardiovascular fitness is the single most important factor in improving your overall physical condition. Yet, it was largely unheard of by the general public until a few years ago. It is the only type of exercise that can *potentially* add years to your life; potentially, because no one can guarantee you a longer life. Your genetic background and family medical history are also major determining factors.

How might cardiovascular fitness prolong your life? Think of your heart as a machine, good for so many beats in a lifetime. Regular cardiovascular exercise reduces the number of heartbeats used per minute during normal activity, rest, and activity. The heart beats less per minute, per hour, per day, and so on. Therefore, theoretically, you are saving up heart beats and should live longer.

An example: Let's say that your heart is good for 2.5 billion heartbeats (a good ballpark figure), and then you are dead. If you have a resting heart rate of 80 beats per minute and a well-conditioned athlete has a heart rate of 60, then you are using up 20 beats more per minute than the athlete—per minute, per hour, per day, etc. Guess who should live longer?

It is ironic that to gain this cardiovascular advantage, we must use up our precious heart beats, at least in a short-term sense. If we have only a limited number of heart beats in a lifetime, it might be tempting to spend our whole lives in bed and/or doing as little as possible to save those valuable heart beats. Yet, if we did so, our resting heart rates would be much higher than those of a conditioned athlete. We could have a heart rate of 100 beats per minute at rest in contrast to a physically active person with one of 60 beats per minute or less.

How do we reduce our heart rates? Only one way—through cardiovascular exercise. Therefore, in a short-term sense, when we take part in physical activity, we do use up some of our precious heart beats. But from a long-term standpoint, through cardiovascular exercise, our heart rate is reduced at all levels of activity. Indeed, exercise physiologists estimate that, by expending 2,000 extra heart beats during a day's exercise session, we can save 10,000 to 30,000 beats over the remainder of the day. Furthermore, a one-beat saving in the resting or average heart rate translates into 1,440 beats per day, or 525,600 beats per year.[1]

How does cardiovascular exercise reduce heart rate? To keep the muscles in good shape, you might do exercises or lift weights. The heart is a muscle too. Its form of exercise is faster beating, induced through strenuous activity. The heart muscle gradually grows stronger, and can push more blood out with each beat. Therefore, it has to beat less often to get your blood around your body. In other words, the heart beats more efficiently when it is in good cardiovascular condition.

There are other reasons for doing cardiovascular exercise. Since oxygen is carried in the blood, it will be distributed more rapidly from your lungs to your heart to all parts of your body. As a result, you will have more energy, faster. There are dual benefits to cardiovascular conditioning because you involve muscles as well. For example, in running you use your leg muscles; in cross-country skiing, your arms and legs, in addition to stimulating the heart, lungs, and circulatory systems. The reverse is not true. When you do muscular exercise, you don't exercise the heart and lungs sufficiently to derive any long-term cardiovascular benefit.

1. *You and Your Heart Rate,* Fitness and Amateur Sport, Government of Canada, Ottawa, 1978.

Physical Activity Readiness Questionnaire (PAR-Q)*

PARTICIPANT IDENTIFICATION

PAR Q & YOU

PAR-Q is designed to help you help yourself. Many health benefits are associated with regular exercise, and the completion of PAR-Q is a sensible first step to take if you are planning to increase the amount of physical activity in your life.

For most people physical activity should not pose any problem or hazard. PAR-Q has been designed to identify the small number of adults for whom physical activity might be inappropriate or those who should have medical advice concerning the type of activity most suitable for them.

Common sense is your best guide in answering these few questions. Please read them carefully and check (√) the ☐ YES or ☐ NO opposite the question if it applies to you.

YES NO

☐ ☐ 1. Has your doctor ever said you have heart trouble?

☐ ☐ 2. Do you frequently have pains in your heart and chest?

☐ ☐ 3. Do you often feel faint or have spells of severe dizziness?

☐ ☐ 4. Has a doctor ever said your blood pressure was too high?

☐ ☐ 5. Has your doctor ever told you that you have a bone or joint problem such as arthritis that has been aggravated by exercise, or might be made worse with exercise?

☐ ☐ 6. Is there a good physical reason not mentioned here why you should not follow an activity program even if you wanted to?

☐ ☐ 7. Are you over age 65 and not accustomed to vigorous exercise?

If You Answered

YES to one or more questions

If you have not recently done so, consult with your personal physician by telephone or in person BEFORE increasing your physical activity and/or taking a fitness test. Tell him what questions you answered YES on PAR-Q, or show him your copy.

programs

After medical evaluation, seek advice from your physician as to your suitability for:
- unrestricted physical activity, probably on a gradually increasing basis.
- restricted or supervised activity to meet your specific needs, at least on an initial basis. Check in your community for special programs or services.

NO to all questions

If you answered PAR-Q accurately, you have reasonable assurance of your present suitability for:
- A GRADUATED EXERCISE PROGRAM - A gradual increase in proper exercise promotes good fitness development while minimizing or eliminating discomfort.
- AN EXERCISE TEST - Simple tests of fitness (such as the Canadian Home Fitness Test) or more complex types may be undertaken if you so desire.

postpone

If you have a temporary minor illness, such as a common cold.

* Developed by the British Columbia Ministry of Health. Conceptualized and critiqued by the Multidisciplinary Advisory Board on Exercise (MABE). Translation, reproduction and use in its entirety is encouraged. Modifications by written permission only. Not to be used for commercial advertising in order to solicit business from the public.
Reference: PAR-Q Validation Report, British Columbia Ministry of Health, 1978.
* Produced by the British Columbia Ministry of Health and the Department of National Health & Welfare.

Figure 1

FITNESS TRAILS AS PART OF THE TOTAL FITNESS PICTURE

Fitness trails must be set up scientifically, following all good general principles of conditioning, if physical improvement is to be achieved by users. Let's review some guidelines for exercise.

GETTING READY TO EXERCISE

Everyone should first consult his or her family physician *before* embarking on a fitness program of any type. This is essential. It is the most important precautionary measure you can take to ensure your physical safety. Ill-advised, ungoverned exercise can be dangerous. Sudden bursts of strenuous activity can be harmful to people who are not in good physical condition.

Many people are needlessly injured when participating in exercise. Much of this could be avoided with a simple medical examination before starting.

Dr. Kenneth Cooper, author of the famous "aerobics" program, suggests that no more than one year should have passed since your last physical and that three months is the limit for those over 35 years of age.[1] Your family doctor should be aware of any medical problems that might restrict your participation, such as a bad back or trick knee. A stress electrocardiogram is a good idea for those over 35 to make sure your heart can withstand the stress of exercise and to help in designing an exercise program for your specific needs. The main purpose of a medical examination is to spot heart, lung, and blood vessel problems that could prove to be potentially dangerous when exercising. Heavy smoking, high blood pressure, obesity, inactivity, high cholesterol, a history of heart disease in the immediate family, and stress are all considerations in how quickly you progress on your exercise program.

Another means by which you may judge whether you are ready to exercise is to complete the Physical Activity Readiness Questionnaire (PAR-Q) that follows. Developed by the British Columbia Ministry of Health and endorsed by the Canadian Department of National Health and Welfare, it has been adopted nationwide as an effective screening device for all individuals wishing to begin an exercise program and/or take a fitness test[2] (see Figure 1).

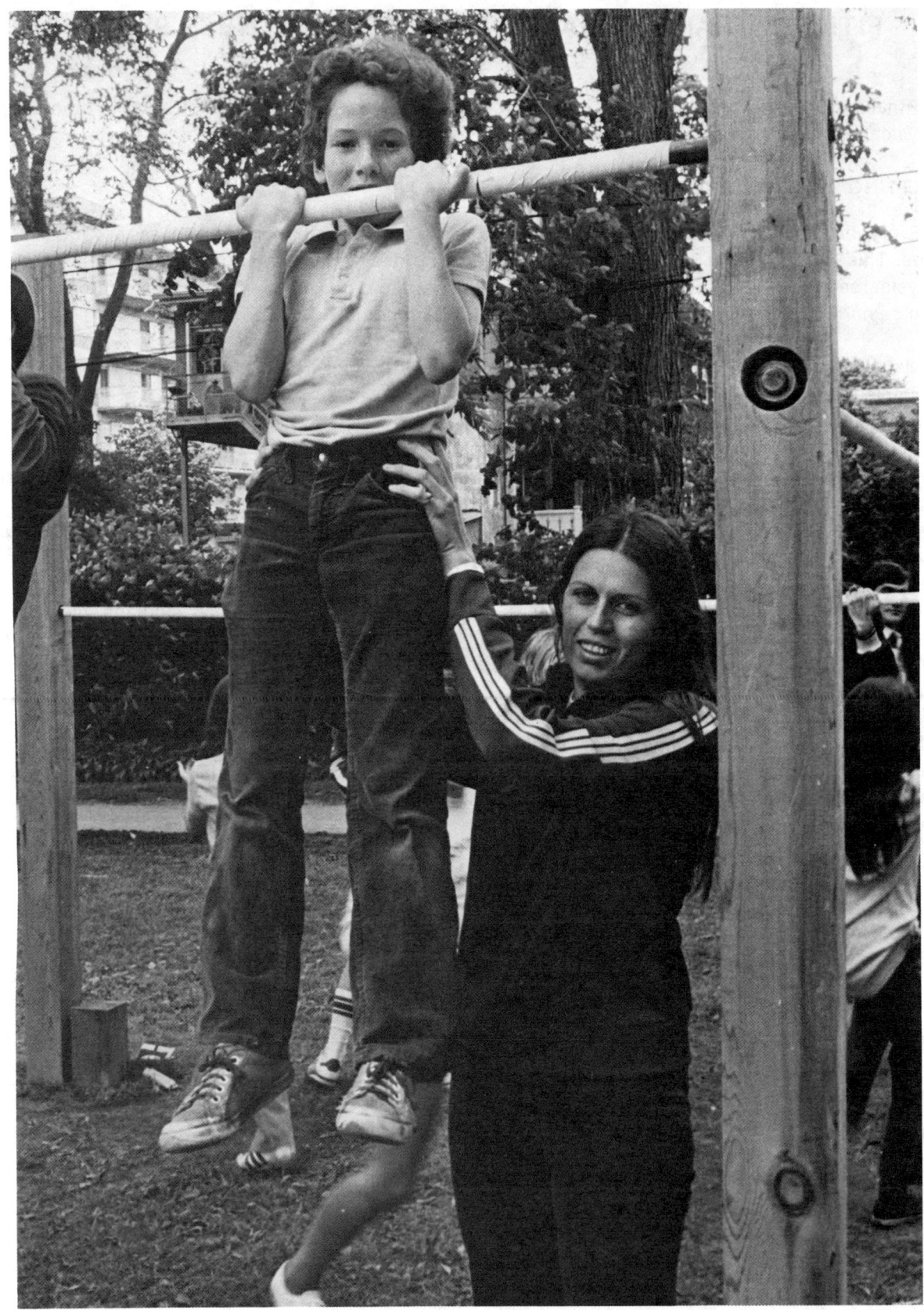

HOW MANY TIMES A WEEK?

The more often you exercise each week, the faster you will become more physically fit. However, research indicates that you should participate a minimum of three or four times a week, letting no more than 48 hours elapse between workouts. Do more if you wish, but not less.

Weekend athletes should pay heed. Exercising infrequently can hurt you more than help improve your physical condition.

Nor can you store up fitness. This means that every week, at least three times a week, you must take part in some form of cardiovascular exercise. Therefore, it is recommended that participants work out at least three to four times a week using a fitness trail in combination with other fitness activities.

Fitness is a lifetime habit. It's easier to maintain than attain.

INCLUDE CARDIOVASCULAR AND MUSCULAR EXERCISE

To be in good overall physical condition, you must exercise all parts of the body—including the heart.

Fitness trails are primarily designed as cardiovascular training circuits, although there is a definite muscle component as well. You run to each exercise station—which improves your cardiovascular condition—and perform the indicated activity when you arrive there—which benefits your muscular condition.

Thus, it is possible to achieve a well-rounded fitness program using a fitness trail.

BUILD UP GRADUALLY

Don't try to do too much too soon. The older you are, the more important this becomes. You cannot ask your body to do as much at age 30 or 40 as it could at 20 years of age. You have lots of time to improve, a lifetime in fact, so take it easy. There's no hurry. Nothing discourages exercise like stiff muscles. Most people do too much too soon, and end up by quitting their fitness programs altogether. You are better off to do a little and keep going, rather than do a lot but stop.

MODERATE SUSTAINED ACTIVITIES

These are preferable to heavy, forceful exercises, particularly for beginners. Brief periods of rest interspersed with activity are invaluable in building up endurance gradually.

A fitness trail fits right in with this concept. You run at your own pace to each exercise station. Then you stop to do the indicated exercise. Of course, you can pause at this time as well to take a breather if you need one.

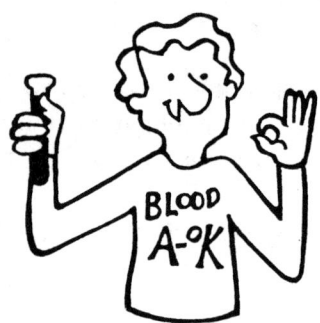

CONSULT A PROFESSIONAL

Look for advice and help from trained personnel with such academic credentials as a degree in physical education or exercise science. Organizations such as the American College of Sports Medicine, the American Board of Fitness Instructors, or the Canadian Association of Sport Sciences also offer courses and accreditation to upgrade the standards in the field.

Most important, follow physical conditioning programs as prescribed. Do not make your own innovations. Professionals are paid to know what they are doing. If you have any problems, consult with them. After all, that's what you are paying them for.

Thus, fitness trails must be set up by fitness professionals following scientific principles such as we are discussing now. This is one more way to ensure the health and physical safety of participants.

EXERCISE AT THE SAME TIME EVERY DAY

Research shows that you are more likely to continue exercising if you set aside a particular time each day and let nothing encroach on it. Think of it as time you are spending on yourself.

WEAR CORRECT CLOTHES AND SHOES

The general rule is that clothing should be light, loose, comfortable, and protective. Shirts should be light and airy to provide good ventilation. In the summer, you want to wear clothes that can breathe, meaning that they allow moisture and heat to escape. Therefore, cotton is your best choice of fabric in shirts. Shorts should be made of nylon and should be loose to prevent chafing of the skin. Cotton shorts should be avoided because they absorb more perspiration than nylon and tend to have bulky seams. Sweatsuits are designed primarily to keep you warm and protect you from the elements so buy them for practicality, not for the way they look. Loose-fitting suits made of cotton, or a combination of cotton and porous synthetic fiber, are best. A hood, pockets, and front zipper are features to consider in sweat tops. Sweatpants should be tight at the ankle.

The choice of shoe can make or break a runner. Yet, until a decade ago, there was very little choice in footwear. A jogger's foot hits the ground about 10,000 times an hour with a force equal to approximately three times the runner's weight. With 125 ligaments, 31 muscles, and 28 bones, is it any wonder that the foot is a prime candidate for injury?

The accepted style for runners is slightly flat-footed, landing heel first. Thus, the heel bears the greatest amount of impact. For this reason, it requires extra cushioning. A heel raise also helps to reduce the strain on the Achilles tendon, which attaches at the heel and runs up the back of the calf. To provide stability on impact, heels should be wide to help distribute the body's weight evenly and prevent ankles from rolling and twisting. Heel cups in shoes should be rigid, made of leather, and should surround the heel, giving added strength to the entire shoe and preventing the heel from lifting out, a common cause of blisters.

The outer part of the shoe, commonly referred to as the "uppers," should be a combination of nylon and leather. Nylon is light, washable, water-resistant, permits air to circulate, and does not crack or become stiff with age or from wetness. Leather reinforcements at the toe and heel give the shoe extra durability.

The sole of the shoe, usually made of rubber, provides cushioning and protection. It should not bend *between* the heel and the ball of the foot. However, it should be very flexible *at* the ball of the foot where it flexes dramatically.

Arch supports are very important in a shoe, and help to prevent foot, leg, and back problems. Good shoes generally supply a build-in arch support.

Since fitness trails require a great deal of running, your best bet is to buy a brand-name shoe made specifically for jogging. Look for "training flats." Try the shoes on in the store, wearing the socks (one or two pairs) you plan to use when running. Lace the shoes snugly and walk around for a few minutes. As for correct size, select shoes that generally conform to the shape of your foot, allowing ½ to ¾ of an inch of extra room at the toe. Check to see that you can't lift your heel out of the back of the shoe and that there are no rough edges or stitching on the inside that might cause cuts or blisters.

Proper footwear and clothes are doubly important on a fitness trail. You are outside facing the elements unprotected, and sudden weather changes can occur. In addition, trail surfaces are not generally very smooth or even. It's easy to twist or sprain an ankle. Thus, it is important to come prepared with correct clothing and shoes. In fact, some doctors claim that injuries could be decreased by 20 percent with a prescreening for tight joints and other abnormalities, and the proper choice of shoes.[3]

FITNESS TRAIL DIARY

NAME: _____

DATE	DISTANCE RUN	FITNESS LEVEL	TIME	RESTING PULSE RATE	PULSE RATE IMMEDIATELY AFTER EXERCISE	WEIGHT

Figure 2

KEEP A PROGRESS CHART

This is an excellent motivational device so that you can see how your physical condition is improving. It might look like Figure 2.

There are many possible factors which can be used to assess your progress. The above are some of the most important. Here's how you should record them.

Date	Each date you use the fitness trail.
Distance run	The distance (in miles or kilometers) of the fitness trail you follow.
Fitness level	Beginner, intermediate, or advanced.
Time	The time it takes to cover the fitness trail pathway selected.
Resting pulse rate	Your lowest pulse/heart rate of the day. This should be taken in the morning, after you wake up, but *before* you get up out of bed. Follow the directions on page 25.
Pulse rate immediately after exercise	This is your *EXERCISE* pulse/heart rate, which should be taken *immediately* after you finish using the fitness trail. Follow the directions on page 25.
Weight	Your true body weight for the day, taken after you get up in the morning, *after* having gone to the bathroom, *before* eating.

When you go through the fitness trail, keep track of the data as listed above. This will help you improve your physical condition and chart your progress. In particular, try to improve your individual time by completing the course in less time. This will happen gradually. Do not expect your running times to decrease drastically every day. It will occur over time, taking at least six weeks to two months at *each* of the three fitness trail levels—beginner, intermediate, and advanced.

The most important indicator that your fitness program is working is your resting pulse rate. If you exercise and use the fitness trail regularly, you should see your resting pulse rate decrease very gradually. This is a very positive sign that your cardiovascular exercise program is achieving results, and that your heart is working more efficiently.

Warm-Up Exercises

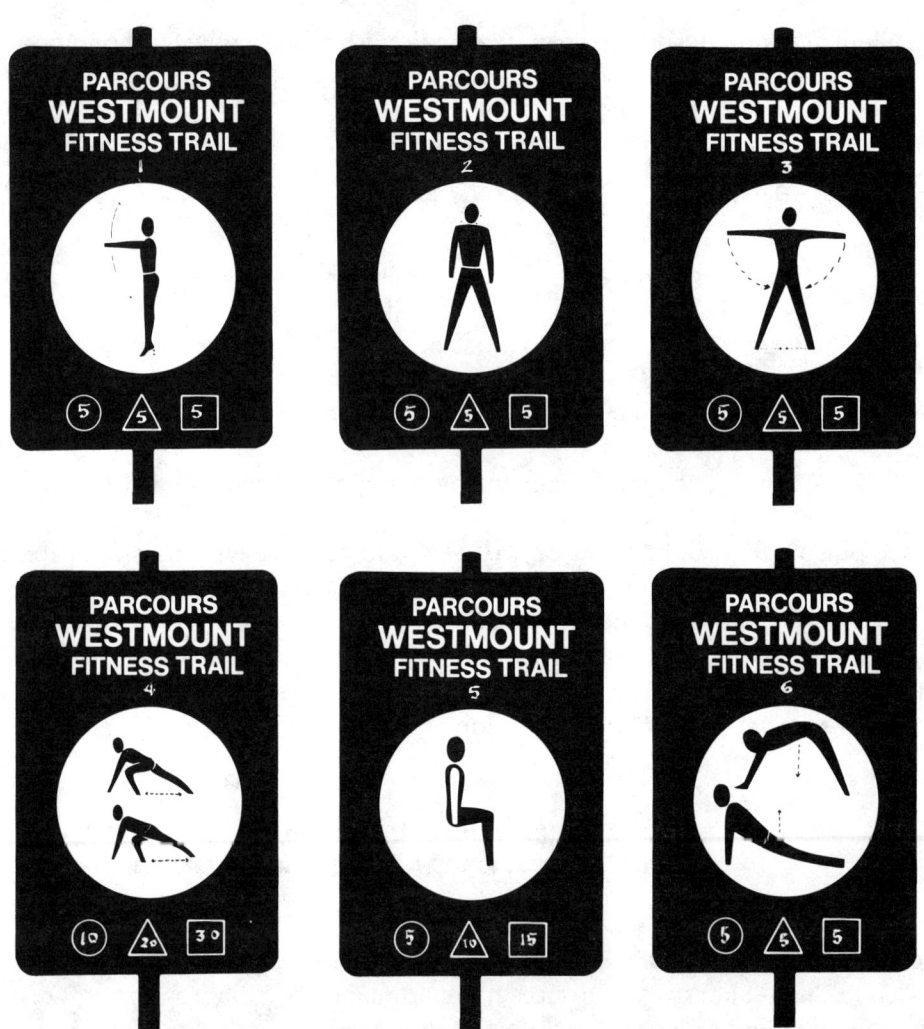

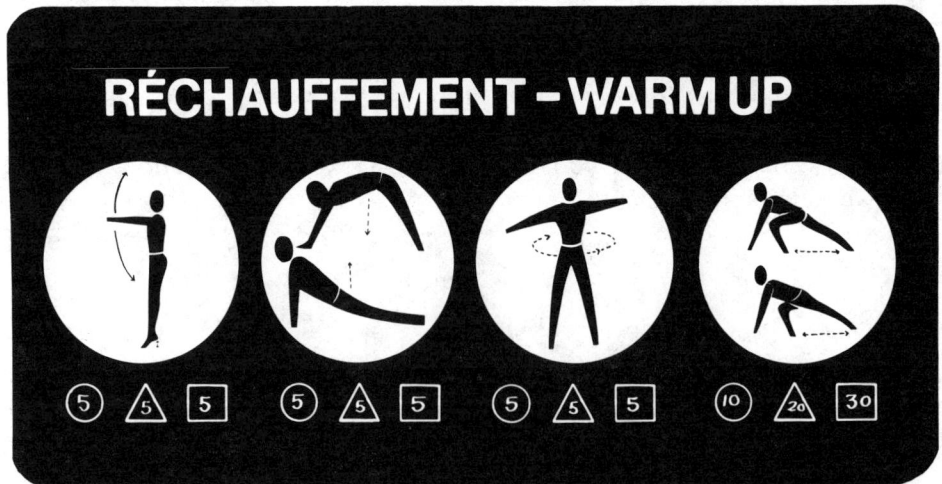

Figure 3

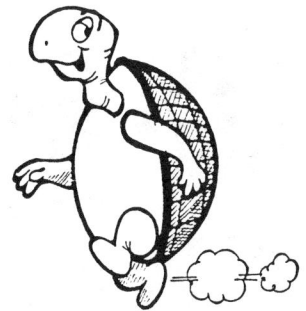

WARM UP GRADUALLY

Sixty percent of athletic injuries could be prevented by training and warming up, according to some sports medicine specialists.[4] Preparing the body for activity helps to ease your heart into more strenuous exercise, and stretches the muscles, helping to prevent later muscle stiffness.

Just as you give your car a chance to warm up in the morning before driving it, so you must do the same for your body before exercising it. A proper warm-up helps prevent injuries like torn muscles and ligaments, strains, pulls, and sprains, as well as helping to reduce stiffening muscles. It also eases that most important muscle, the heart, gently into the more vigorous demands of exercise and gives it a chance to gradually adjust to higher workloads.

To be most effective, the warm-up should include whole-body activities that raise muscle and blood temperature enough to produce slight sweating or a "glow" without causing undue fatigue, as this is just the beginning of your workout.

The idea is to begin slowly and gradually progress to the more vigorous actions of the exercise or sport you are to perform. To a large extent, your warm-up should consist of *stretching,* which should be done *slowly,* with *no bouncing.* Stretching positions should be *held from 20 to 60 seconds* for each repetition, and of course, you must warm up *all* parts of the body. Remember—the idea is to stretch gently with no sharp, quick, static motions. Finally, incorporate an easy jog, building up gradually to a run.

Other general rules for warming up:

1. Never overstretch or you defeat the whole point of a warm-up which is to prevent injury, not to cause it. Exert yourself when stretching, but never go to the point of pain.
2. Do not hold your breath during a warm-up or exercise program. If you have problems, exhale on exertion.
3. The harder the main activity, the more important the warm-up.
4. The more unfit the person, the more important the warm-up.
5. The harder the main activity, the longer the warm-up should be.

Thus, all fitness trails must make provision for warm-up exercises. This can be done in two ways. If the fitness trail is 1½ miles or more, it is possible to schedule a warm-up over the first six exercise stations. For shorter fitness trails, a warm-up station can be located at the start, before the first exercise station. Samples of both may be seen in Figure 3.

17

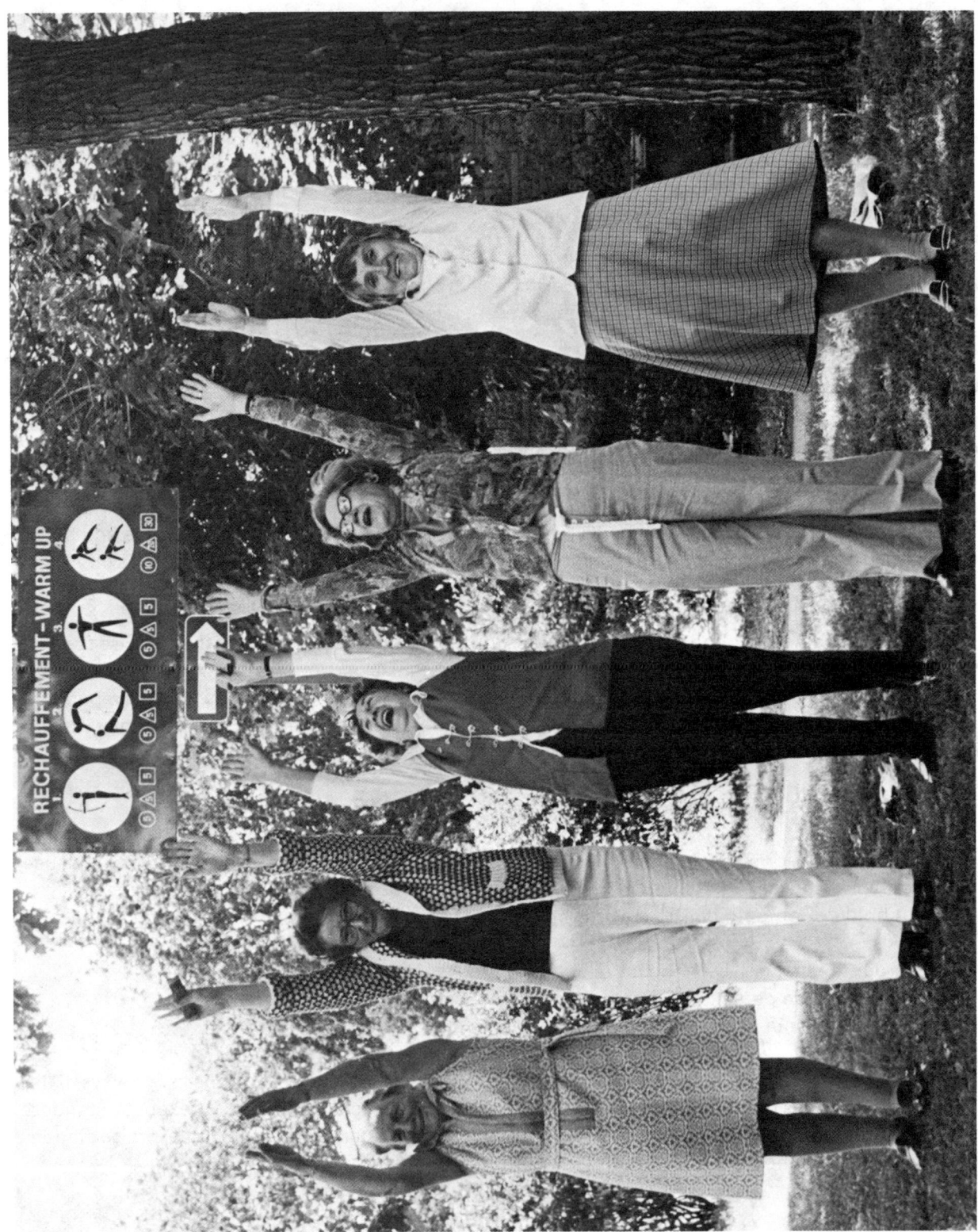

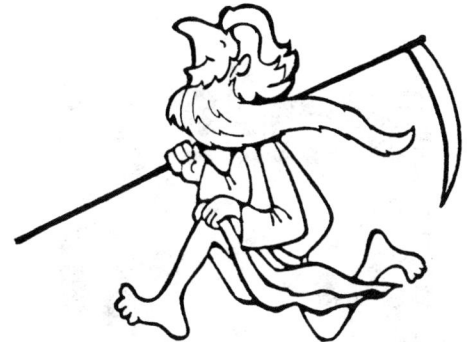

DON'T OVEREXERT

Once you have started to exercise, don't strain yourself. Signs of overexertion are pain in the chest, breathlessness, dizziness, and nausea. If you experience any of these symptoms, stop your exercise immediately. If any of them persist, consult a doctor. If not, in the future reduce the intensity or duration of your activity.

Remember that you should never feel pain when exercising. Aching and stiff muscles are an indication that you are working too hard. On the other hand, while not overexerting, you must ensure that you exercise strenuously enough that you do improve your physical condition over time. You get out of exercise what you put into it. No one and no machine can do the work for you. Thus, there is a midway point between participating so vigorously that you feel pain, and doing so little that you are wasting your time.

TO IMPROVE, "OVERLOAD"

Once you have realized some results, to continue improving your physical condition you must "overload." The overload principle states that your body will gradually adapt to any level of activity. For continued improvement you must then do more, that is, "overload."

For example, let's say that you are at the beginner level of the fitness trail program. At one exercise station, novices are supposed to do five repetitions. At first, this seems hard but in time you find it easier. To improve further at this exercise station, you must then do more, that is, increase the number of repetitions. Increasing the intensity in this manner is known as "overloading," which you continue to do until you have reached your desired fitness level.

Both cardiovascular and muscular exercise require overloading to bring about improvement. In your progress chart (see Figure 2), it was suggested that you gradually increase the intensity of the running you do between each exercise station, thus decreasing the time in which you complete the entire fitness trail. This is, in essence, overloading. Increasing the number of repetitions you do at each exercise station over a period of time, as described above, is the way to improve the condition of the muscles. This is built into the fitness trail program by providing three levels of participation—beginner, intermediate, and advanced.

Cool Down Exercises

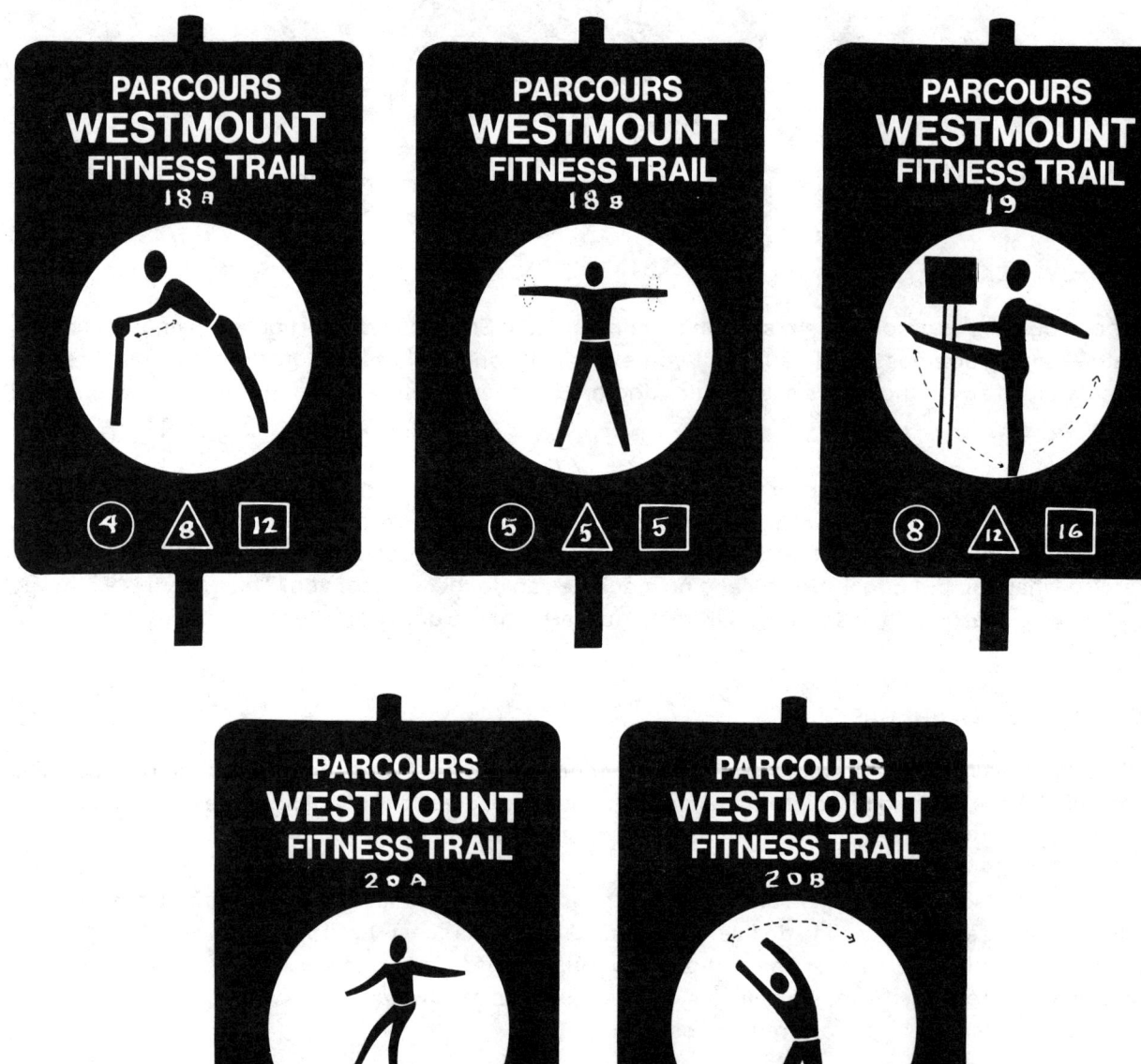

Figure 4

When two exercises (A and B) are provided at any given exercise station, as can be seen above, "A" exercises are to be used in the summer when it is possible to use equipment; "B" exercises are for use in the winter when equipment is buried under snow.

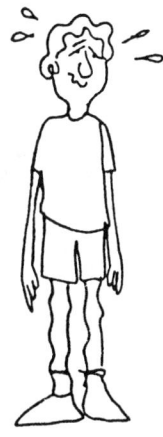

COOL-DOWN

Just as important as the warm-up is cooling down after exercise. The latter allows the body to adjust from the exercise to resting state, permitting recovery from the stress of the exercise. Activities of diminishing intensity permit the return of circulation and various body functions to preexercise levels.

It is very tempting to forget about tapering off gradually. Instead, one ends exercise abruptly by sitting or lying down. This can be very dangerous. The blood may not be returned as quickly to the heart as it is being pumped out. The heart may then be left beating on an almost empty chamber. At the very least, dizziness or faintness may result; shock is also a possibility. Among older adults, heart attacks may occur.

To allow the body to gradually readjust to a resting state, whole-body activities, stretches, and gentle relaxation exercises aid the venous return of blood to the heart and the restoration of normal blood circulation. They also facilitate the dissipation of body heat produced during strenuous activity, and aid in the elimination of lactic acid, the substance which causes the muscles to tire and ache.

Therefore, it is vital to include a cool-down as an integral part of any fitness trail. It should continue over several stations at the end until the pulse rate has fallen below at least 120 beats per minute and profuse sweating has stopped. This will require a minimum of ten minutes.

Figure 4 presents a sample cool-down for your fitness trail.

FINAL ENCOURAGEMENT

Don't get discouraged. The first ten weeks of any fitness program are the hardest. That's when you will suffer through tiredness, blisters, sore muscles, etc. The important thing is that you are on your way to a fit body. You didn't get out of shape overnight, so remember—it takes time to improve. Stick with it. Your fit body will be worth it.

ENDNOTES

1. Kenneth H. Cooper, *The Aerobics Way,* Bantam, New York, 1977, p. 52.

2. British Columbia Ministry of Health, *PAR-Q Validation Report,* May 1978.

3. "Woes of the Weekend Jock," *Time,* August 21, 1978, p. 50.

4. Ibid.

PULSE RATE-BASED FITNESS PROGRAMS

Measuring your heart rate or pulse rate is an effective way to monitor your progress in the cardiovascular portion of your fitness program. Remember that heart rate and pulse rate are basically the same thing. Only the measurement location is different. You take your heart rate just as it says—at your heart—using a stethoscope, while your pulse can be measured at the wrist, throat, or on the temple.

Heart/pulse rate can provide you with a great deal of information about the condition of your body. American author Dr. Laurence Morehouse says that the pulse is nothing more nor less than an accurate index of how many times the heart is beating against the column of blood in your circulatory vessels.

> It informs you of every change that is taking place in your person. It tells you if your body temperature is rising, or if you're cooling down. It tells you how fast you're burning up energy and using oxygen from the air. It tells you how your body is handling the chemical wastes in your blood. It tells you how your muscles are involved and working. It even tells you about the state of your emotions and attitudes. It pulls all of these together, weighs them and comes out with a single signal that reports your overall condition.[1]

Therefore, you could call your pulse rate your "built-in computer," as it gives you important information about the condition of your body.

Many factors can affect your heart/pulse rate. Age is one. Your maximum rate decreases as you get older, while at rest it stays relatively stable throughout adulthood.

Gender also affects heart rate. Men generally have a lower rate than women, and boys lower than girls. This is due to the reduced oxygen-carrying capabilities of the female's circulatory system.

A normal heart rate for a man is between 60 and 80 beats per minute, and for a woman, between 65 and 85. An average heart rate for boys is approximately 80-84 beats per minute and 82-89 beats per minute for girls. However, as mentioned, many factors determine your heart rate.

The fitter you are, the lower your heart rate. Well-conditioned athletes, male or female, may have resting heart rates of less than 50 beats per minute. When you are asleep your heart rate is lower than at any other time of the day. When you awaken, it increases five to ten beats per minute. Your pulse rate increases gradually during the day, affected by such things as tension, anxiety, caffeine, food, air temperature, nicotine, alcohol, exercise, and your normal daily activities, and will be another five to ten beats higher by the time you go to bed.

Increases in heat and humidity can increase a normal heart rate, as can the presence of a fever in your body. Heart rate increases approximately 20 beats per minute for every rise of 1 degree centigrade above normal body temperature.

Smokers have higher heart rates than nonsmokers because nicotine, even in small amounts, raises the heart rate. Carbon monoxide produced from tobacco smoke also creates this effect. Similarly, substances containing caffeine artificially raise the heart rate. Most of you know that it can be found in tea and coffee, but did you know that caffeine is present in varying amounts in soft drinks and cocoa?

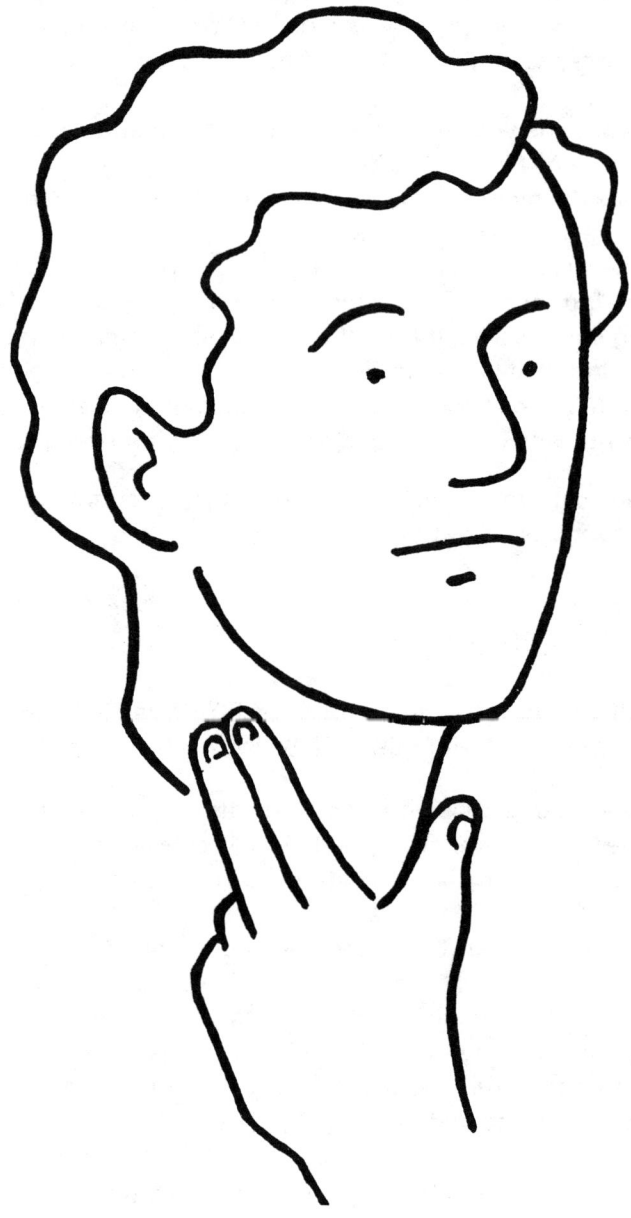

Figure 5

Why should you be concerned with your heart rate? Recent studies have indicated that "resting heart rates of 80 and greater were associated with sizable increases in risk of dying over the next ten years from all causes, all cardiovascular-renal diseases, coronary heart disease, and sudden death."[2]

Pulse rate is a very individual index of your general well-being. Therefore, if you do not conform to the norms specified here, do not be overly alarmed. However, if your pulse rate is excessively high all the time, you should consult your family doctor. Of course, the lower your pulse rate is, generally speaking, the better it is. A low pulse rate indicates that your heart is beating more efficiently and has to beat less often during rest, exercise, or normal activity. The heart then has a chance to take a longer rest between beats and it fills up more slowly and completely.

Paradoxically, the best way to lower your pulse rate is to make it beat faster for short periods of exercise. This strengthens the heart so it can perform more efficiently at lower rates.

Your pulse/heart rate is one of the most easily accessible means to evaluate both how hard you are exercising, and how well you are responding to your cardiovascular exercise program. If you keep a record of your exercise pulse rate, as was suggested earlier, you should see a gradual decrease in your pulse rate. This, of course, assumes that you also exercise regularly, at least three to four times a week, approximately 30 minutes each workout.

A minimum of six weeks to two months is required before there is any noticeable change. This decrease in pulse rate is one means by which you can determine that your cardiovascular exercise program is working.

HOW TO TAKE YOUR RESTING PULSE RATE

1. Before rising in the morning, do the following:

2. Find your pulse on your throat using the *fingers only* of one hand. Your pulse can be located directly under the chin on either side of the neck. (You can also take your pulse at the wrist. The throat pulse is usually easier to find.)

3. Count your pulse for 15 seconds and multiply by 4. This is your resting pulse rate.

HOW TO TAKE YOUR EXERCISE PULSE RATE

1. Stop exercising.

2. Follow steps 2 and 3 as above.

NOTE: It is very important to take your pulse rate *immediately* after exercise to get a true reading.

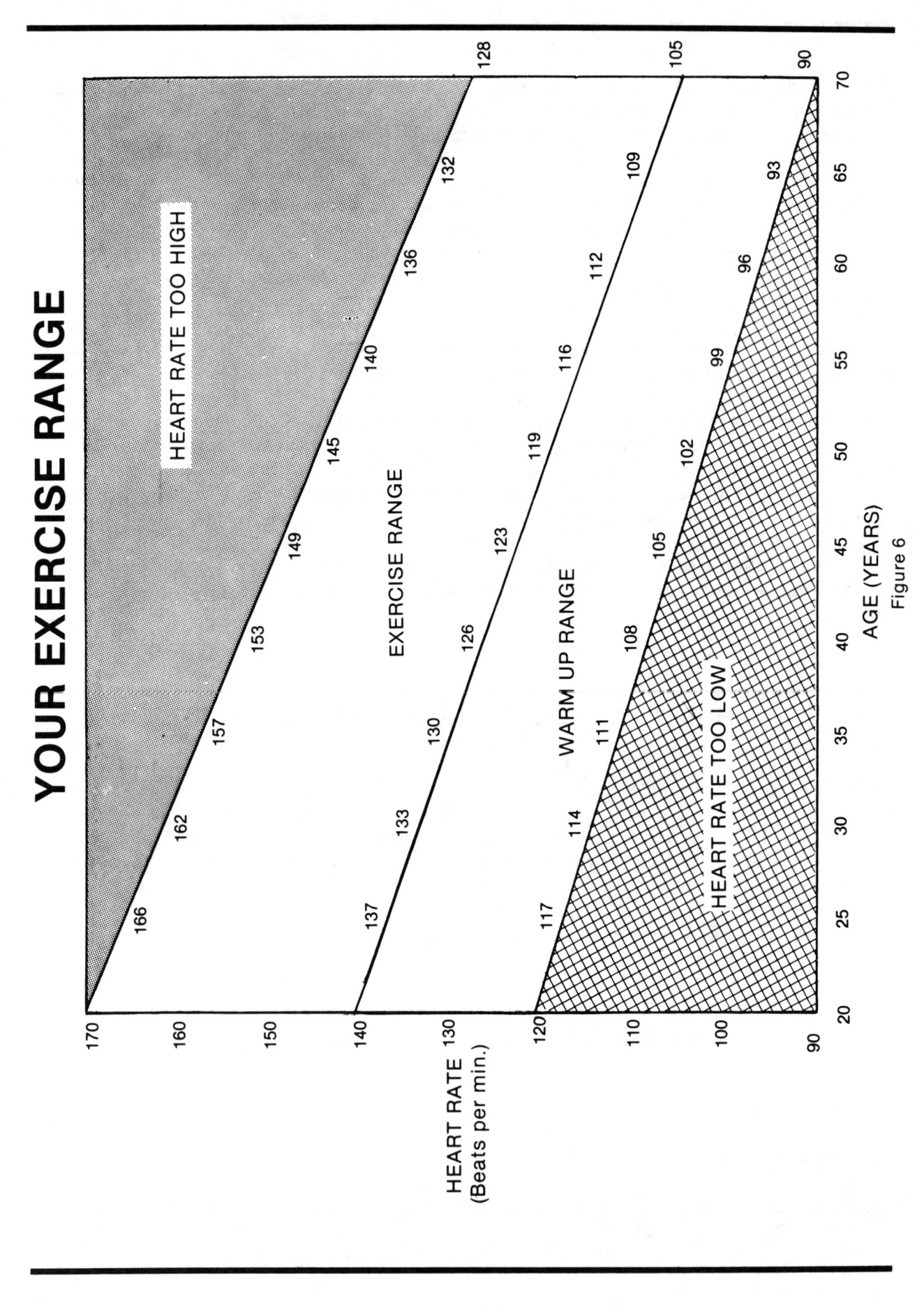
Figure 6

HOW HARD SHOULD YOU EXERCISE?

A reliable indicator of the intensity of exercise is your heart/pulse rate. As it increases, so does the intensity of the activity.

As a general rule, your exercise pulse rate should fall within a range of 70 to 85 percent of your maximum heart rate. This is called your "exercise" or aerobic" range.

When participating in cardiovascular activity of any type, you should attempt to stay within this range. Higher than this and you are running risks; lower and you will not see any improvement in your physical condition.

There are several ways to determine your aerobic range. One easy method is to subtract your age from 200 to give you your upper limit, and subtract your age from 170 for your lower limit. For example, if you are 40 years of age: 200 - 40 = 160; 170 - 40 = 130. Therefore, when exercising, 40-year-olds must increase their pulse rates to at least 130 beats per minute during exercise if they are to obtain any long-term cardiovascular benefit, and should not exceed 160 beats per minute, or it could be dangerous.

Another simple way to establish your exercise or aerobic range is to consult Figure 6. Heart rate measured in beats per minute is listed on the left-hand side of the chart; age can be found on the bottom. Find your age group, then read up the chart to determine the upper and lower limits of your aerobic heart beat range.

WHY IS YOUR EXERCISE/AEROBIC RANGE SO IMPORTANT?

Many people make the mistake of working themselves too hard when they exercise—much harder than they have to to become physically fit. On the other hand, others don't work hard enough and never become as fit as they should be.

The dilemma, then, is how hard should you exercise to ensure that you receive cardiovascular benefit, and at the same time prevent yourself from overworking and hurting yourself?

The answer is quite simple. For maximum benefit and for prevention of injury, keep your exercise heart/pulse rate within your "exercise" or "aerobic" range.

Note that, as people grow older, they don't have to work themselves as hard as young people to reach the same cardiovascular fitness level. For instance, if you look at Figure 6, you will see that the bottom of the exercise range for a 20-year-old is 140 beats per minute. Yet, this is the top of the exercise range for a 55-year-old. Too many older people ignore such physiological restraints of their bodies. They push themselves much too hard, much harder than they should or have to. And this could be dangerous.

CONCLUSION: *Keep your heart/pulse rate in the exercise range designated for your age group.* Be safe, not foolish!

FITNESS TRAILS AND PULSE RATE-BASED EXERCISE

Fitness trails are primarily cardiovascular programs, although muscular activity is incorporated through the various exercise stations. Thus, when using a fitness trail, remember to keep your pulse rate within the upper and lower ranges designated for your particular age group, as you would for any fitness activity.

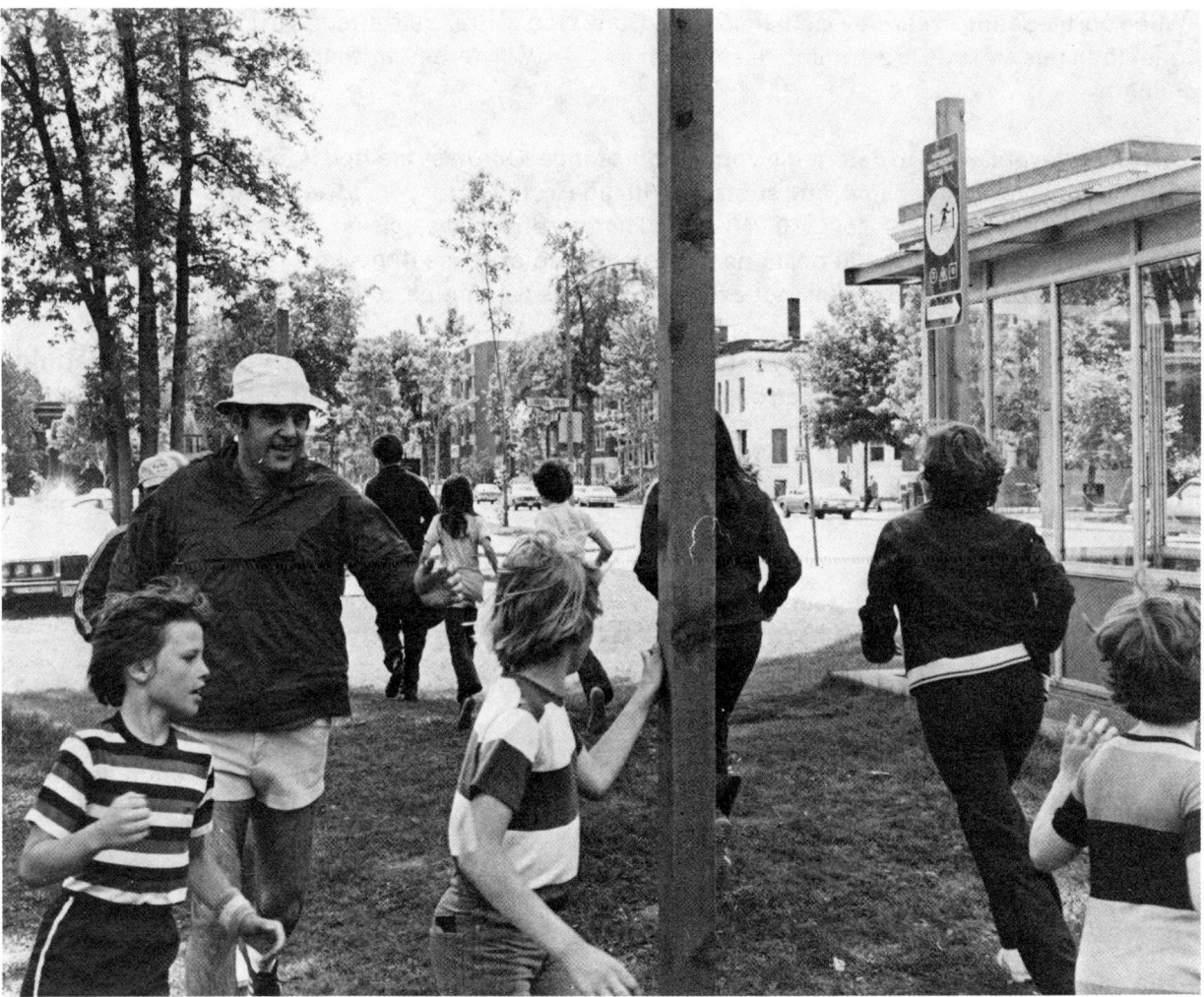

ENDNOTES

1. Laurence E. Morehouse and Leonard Gross, *Total Fitness in 30 Minutes a Week,* Simon and Schuster, New York, 1975, p. 131.

2. Stamler et al, *Peoples Gas Company Study,* in *You and Your Heart Rate,* Fitness and Amateur Sport, Government of Canada, Ottawa, 1978.

HOW TO SET UP A FITNESS PROGRAM

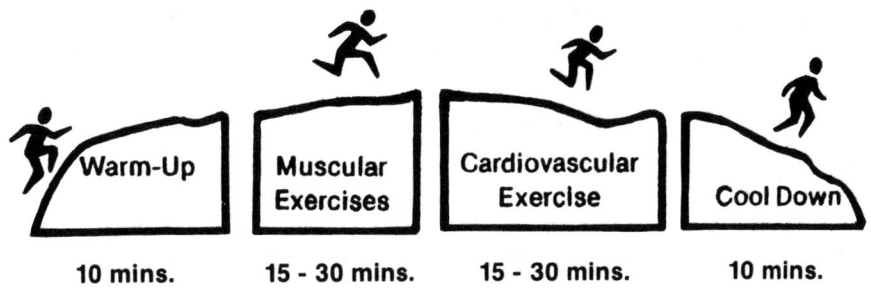

All exercise programs follow the same basic format. This can be built into the layout of the fitness trail, ensuring a safe and effective program.

Regardless of what exercise regime you follow, you should always *warm up*. This is the first part of any workout. Basically you are preparing your body for exercise.

Phase two is the main body of your fitness program. Here you include both *cardiovascular and muscular exercise.*

Finally, every fitness program should taper off with a *cool-down.* Just as you gradually worked your body up to the exercise phase, so you must give it an opportunity to slowly return to a resting state.

Warming up and cooling down should each take approximately 10 to 15 minutes, while the exercise phase of your fitness program should be at least one-half hour.

This rough outline should serve as a guideline to you when setting up your fitness trail. The progression through the exercise stations follows exactly this same pattern—*WARM UP-EXERCISE (Cardiovascular and Muscular)-COOL DOWN.*

These are the basics of a good conditioning program.

A FITNESS TRAIL FOR EVERYONE

To ensure use by a great number of people, a fitness trail must accommodate not only those in good physical condition, but those in poor and intermediate stages of fitness as well.

Provision of three levels of fitness is suggested: beginner, intermediate, and advanced. Using the symbols of a circle ⑩, triangle △₂₀, and square ▢30 is one simple means. The number of repetitions for each level of fitness condition are marked within these symbols, thus clearly indicating to participants goals for which they may strive.

No matter how you decide to indicate the repetitions at each exercise station, it should be stressed that these are only guidelines. Participants should do as many repetitions as they can without unduly straining themselves. A commonsense approach is best. One of the beauties of a fitness trail is that everyone can do his or her own thing. No one is watching or checking. No one knows or cares what anyone else does. The onus is on the individual. Everyone does his or her best. Competition is against oneself.

Three levels of participation (beginner, intermediate, advanced) also means that an "overload" can be built into a fitness trail. In other words, by providing these progressively more difficult levels of activity, which gradually increase the suggested number of repetitions for each exercise, individuals must improve their physical condition. This is the ultimate goal of any fitness program.

STEPS IN CONSTRUCTING A FITNESS TRAIL

1. Design the fitness trail. Consult with experts to decide the following: the exercises to be done at each exercise station; the order of these exercises; the number of repetitions for beginners, intermediate, and advanced levels of activity; the pathway for the trail; etc.

2. Choose the fitness trail site. If necessary, obtain permission to construct it there.

3. Select and design equipment to be constructed at the exercise stations that require it.

4. Design the fitness trail signs and have them printed.

5. Determine building materials, tools, and equipment required to construct the fitness trail. Obtain as much as possible for free. Rent or buy the rest.

6. Look into insurance for the fitness trail in case of participant injury.

7. Raise money—set up a budget for the fitness trail.

8. Construct the fitness trail. Install signs and exercise station equipment where required.

9. Provide an opening ceremony with local media and officials invited.

10. Follow up: send brochures to all local groups that might be interested in using the fitness trail, e.g., schools, health clubs, YMCAs, etc.

11. Arrange for seasonal maintenance, e.g., changing signs, repairs, etc.

CONSULTANTS TO DESIGN AND CONSTRUCT THE FITNESS TRAIL

Many people in your community will be interested in supporting this project. Take advantage of their expertise and help.

Contact some of these groups for help.

1. Consult physical education and fitness specialists, YMCAs, community recreation departments, *reputable* fitness clubs (i.e., people who know what they are doing in fitness) to help decide what exercises to do and the repetitions for beginning, intermediate, and advanced participants.

2. Local town engineers, forestry departments, or architectural firms could help in the physical layout of the trail.

3. College departments of forestry, recreation, physical education, and engineering could help in the development and construction of the trail.

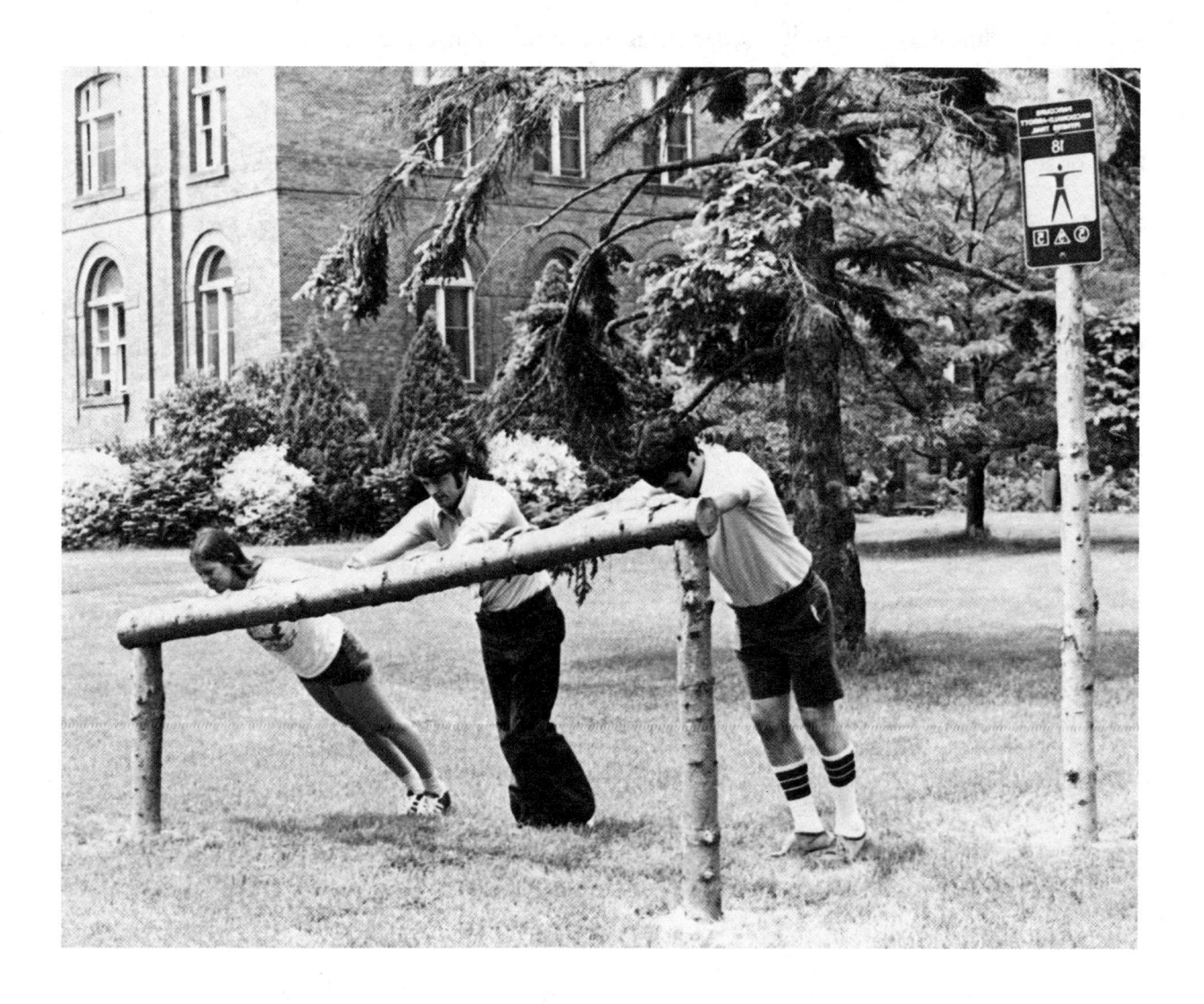

FITNESS TRAIL DESIGN
GENERAL LAYOUT

A fitness trail is generally 1 to 2 miles long with 10 to 20 exercise stations spread throughout.

The exercise stations are designed in a careful progression with warm-up exercises at the first stations, more strenuous exercises following, ending with cool-down exercises for the remaining stations.

Any apparatus that is necessary is right there, built out of logs in keeping with the surrounding scenery; for example, chin-up bars, sit-up platforms. The equipment has been adapted for all ages and heights and sex. Therefore, several people of varying sizes can use the apparatus simultaneously.

A fitness trail with 20 exercise stations might be designed like this:

Warm-Up Exercises - Exercise Stations 1 to 6

These are nonapparatus stations placed about 300 to 400 feet apart. The distances between the warm-up exercises are short.

Exercise Stations 7 to 9

These are more difficult exercises placed about 400 to 500 feet apart.

Exercise Stations 10 and 11

These are less active exercises to serve as a break for participants. Stations are placed about 500 to 700 feet apart. A short circuit might also begin here for a shortened course which eliminates the most strenuous exercises for those who are not in such good shape, or for the old or extremely young.

Exercise Stations 12 to 16

These are the most strenuous exercises. If possible, try to locate them in a shady area, e.g., in a woods. Stations are placed 500 to 700 feet apart.

Cool-Down Exercises - Exercise Stations 17 to 20

These are exercises which allow the body to gradually ease up and relax without coming to a complete stop. During this phase, exercises could be used that work on other aspects of motor performance besides strength, endurance, and flexibility, such as balance. The short circuit should rejoin the fitness trail at Station 17 so that participants can benefit from the cool-down exercises.

EXERCISE STATIONS

The addition of appropriate exercises makes the fitness trail a complete fitness program. Careful consideration must be given as to what exercises and equipment to include and how many repetitions should be done at each fitness level.

1. All exercise stations should be located to the side of the jogging circuit so they do not impede other participants who are running by.
2. Exercise stations located on elevations can be placed closer together than those on flat surfaces.
3. Certain equipment located at exercise stations may permit more than one exercise to be performed. For instance, chin-ups or body circles could both be done on a chin-up bar. (See Exercise "i"). Put signs up for both exercises for the benefit of regular users of the fitness trail, giving them a choice of exercises and thus adding a little variety to the trail.
4. Involve all major muscle groups—trunk and hip, stomach and back, arm and shoulder, neck, leg and knee, and ankle and foot.
5. Do not use the same muscle groups at two consecutive exercise stations, e.g., station 2—sprinter's drill (legs), station 3—log jump (legs).
6. All aspects of muscular exercise should be developed using the fitness trail, e.g., strength, flexibility, endurance, coordination, balance, agility.

A SAMPLE SET OF EXERCISES FOR A FITNESS TRAIL

A. WARM-UP EXERCISES — see Figure 3. These can be done in summer and winter.

B. STRENUOUS EXERCISES
   1. **FOR SUMMER USE ONLY**-using equipment.

   a. Sit-Ups
   With feet anchored under the support and knees bent, lie back. Interlace your fingers behind your head, then sit up. Return to the starting position. This is one count.
   Repetitions: 5-10-15 times

   NOTE: 5 times for beginners
   10 times for intermediates
   15 times for advanced

   b. Chest Raises
   Anchor heels under the support, lying face down, hands behind the head. Raise head, shoulders, chest, and arms as high off the supports as possible. Return to the starting position. This is one count.
   Repetitions: 10-13-16 times

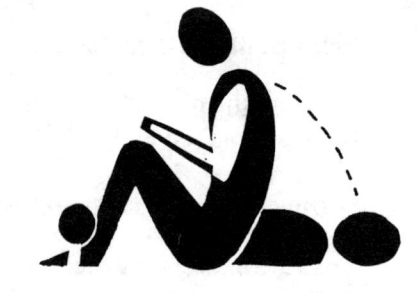

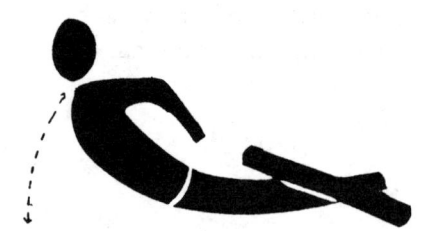

   NOTE: Sit-ups and chest raises can be done on the same piece of equipment at the same exercise station.

c. Step-Ups

Step up onto log with right leg; follow with left. Step down with right leg; follow with left. This is one count.

Repetitions: 10-15-20 times

d. Hurdler's Drill

Put heel of one foot into the heel cup cut into the wooden support. Stand erect. Then try to bend over and touch toe with fingers while gently trying to touch your forehead to your knee. Do not bounce. Return to starting position. This is one count.

Repetitions: 5 times on each knee

e. Sergeant's Jump

Standing under the wooden supports, you will see numbers underneath indicating the various heights. See how high you can jump by seeing the closest number you can touch. The number represents the height you jumped in feet. This is one count.

Repetitions: 5-10-15 times

f. Handwalk

Grasp bars and jump up until you are supported by your arms. Walk along the bar this way, moving one hand at a time. This is one length.

Repetitions: 1-3-5 times doing the length of the equipment

g. Dips

Grasp bars and jump up until you are supported by your arms. Lower body slowly as low as you can go still being able to raise yourself again. Raise body until arms are straight. This is one count.

Repetitions: 2-5-10 times

NOTE: Handwalk and Dips can be done on the same piece of equipment.

h. Body Circles

Grasp bar so your palms face you, feet off the ground. Keep legs together. Swing feet and body in circles. One 360° rotation is one count.

Repetitions: 3-6-10 times each way, left and right

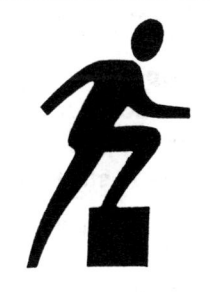

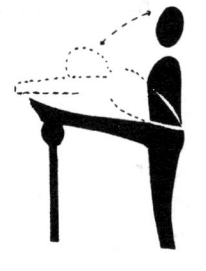

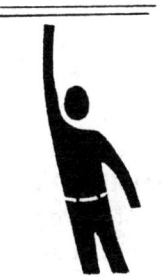

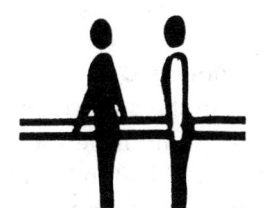

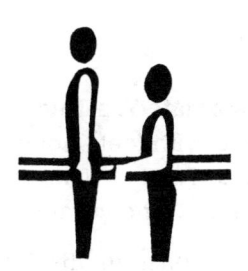

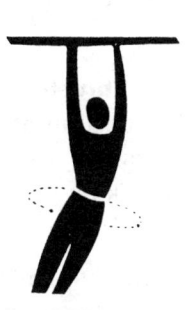

i. Chin-Ups

Grasp bar so your palms face you, feet off the ground, arms straight. Pull your body up by using your arms so that your chin is over the bar. Return to the starting position. This is one count.

Repetitions: 2-4-8 times

NOTE: Body Circles and Chin-Ups can be done on the same piece of equipment.

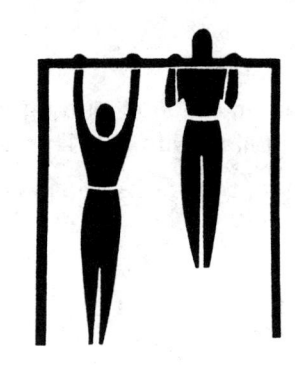

j. Log Jump

Stand on one side of the log, erect with feet together. Hop to the other side of the log with feet still together. This is one count. Continue down the log.

Repetitions: 10-15-20 times. 1 count per hop

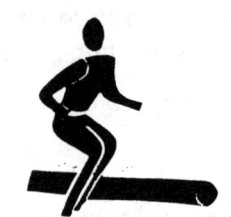

2. FOR SUMMER OR WINTER USE—The following exercises can be done on foot or wearing cross-country skis. No equipment can be used in the winter because it becomes buried in the snow.

k. Sprinter's Drill

Squat in the starting position for a runner, arms out in front straight, hands on floor, left leg bent and right leg extended back. Reverse position of feet in bouncing movement, bringing right foot to hands, extending left leg back—all in one motion. This is one count.

Repetitions: 10-20-30 times

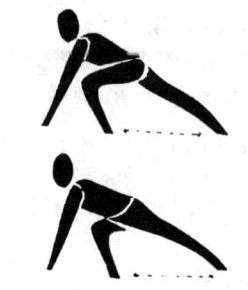

l. Alternate Toe Touch

Stand with feet shoulder-width apart with arms above head at a 45° angle. Twist at waist to right, touch right toe with left hand. Repeat to the left. Concentrate on stretching slowly, not on speed.

Repetitions: 10-15-20 times. Count 1 each time you touch your toe

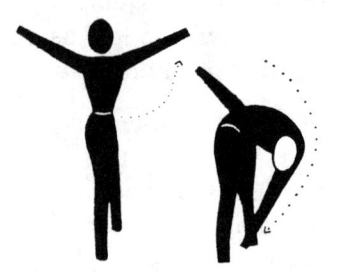

m. Squat Thrusts (Burpies)

Stand erect, arms at sides. Drop to a squatting position, placing hands on the ground. Taking weight on arms, extend legs and feet fully out to the rear (like a push-up position). Return to the squatting position. Stand up. This is one count.

Repetitions: 10-15-20 times

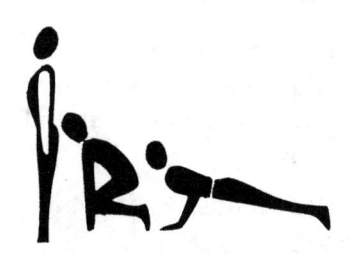

n. Hollowing the Back

Get on your hands and knees with your hands directly under your shoulders and your knees directly under your hips. Tighten your abdominals, tuck your head down, and slowly hump your back like a cat. Hold it. Now slowly relax your back, letting it sink down until it is arched. Look upwards as you do this, and point your posterior up.

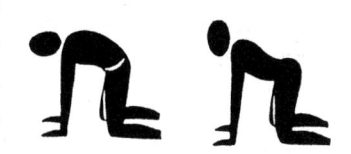

Repetitions: 6-8-10 times

o. Side Leg Raises with Arm Support

Standing to one side of the sign post, hold onto it with one hand. Without moving the upper body, lift the outside leg to the side as high as it will go without forcing it. Lower the leg. This is one count. Alternate legs.

Repetitions: 10-20-30 times on each leg

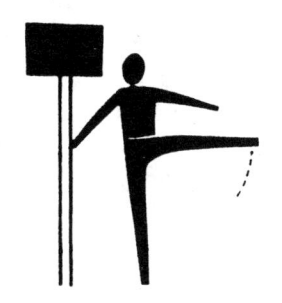

p. Back Arch

Sit on the ground with hands resting behind the hips on the ground. Lift hips off the ground, arch back, and drop head with weight on hands and heels.

Repetitions: 10-15-20 times. Up and down is one count

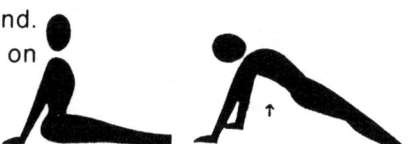

q. Shuttle Run

Stand at one post, touching it with one hand. Run to the other post as fast as you can. This is one count.

Repetitions: 3-6-10 times doing the distance between posts

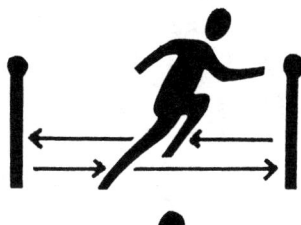

r. Knee-High Running

Bring your knees up high so they touch your hands, which are outstretched from your waist.

Repetitions: 10-20-30 times. 1 count per step

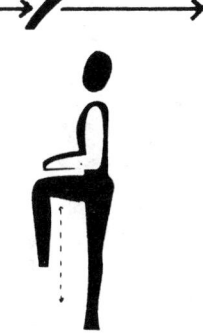

s. Inchworm

Stand erect, arms at sides, feet together. Bend over and touch the floor with finger tips. Slowly walk out on hands until you reach a push-up position. Then walk back up again. This is one count. Try to increase the distance you walk out each time.

Repetitions: 5 times. Out and in is one count

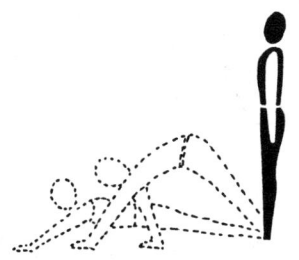

t. Back Kicks

Standing to one side of the sign post, hold onto it with one hand. Lift one leg backwards as far as it can go without forcing it. This is one count. Alternate legs.

Repetitions: 8--16-20 times. 1 count per leg

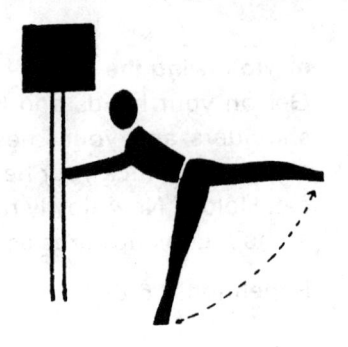

C. **COOL-DOWN EXERCISES**—see Figure 4. Inclined arm push-ups and balance beam can only be done in the summer. Arm circles, leg swings and side bending can be done all year.

Figure 7

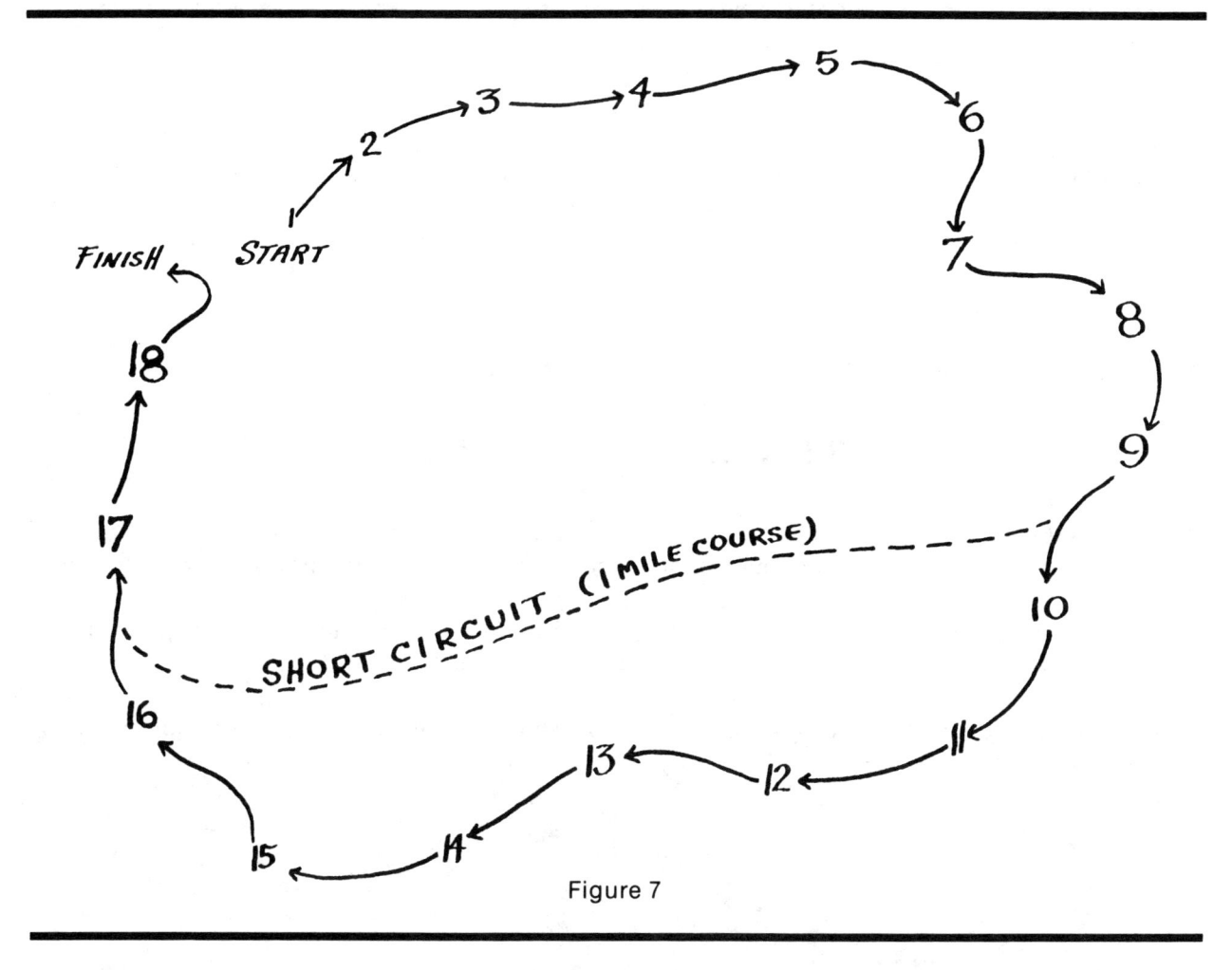

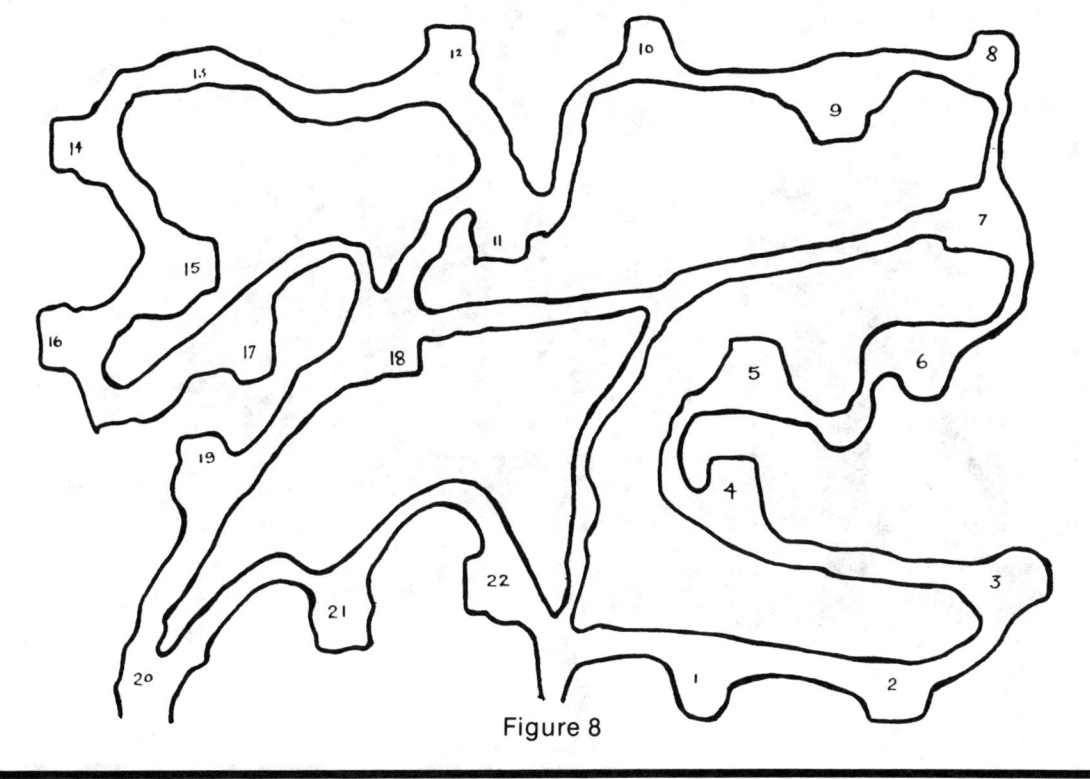

Figure 8

SHORT CIRCUITS

To adapt the trail for use by people of all ages and levels of physical condition, a shorter course of 1 mile or less can be incorporated, for participants who cannot complete the entire fitness trail at first. A short circuit cutting through the middle of your trail, which eliminates the more strenuous exercises, will enable people to build up their physical condition gradually and will encourage its use by senior citizens and very young children who might otherwise be excluded. See Figure 7.

A series of looped trails will also serve the same purpose. See Figure 8.

WINTER FITNESS TRAILS

Fitness trails should be open summer and winter to be practical for most North American situations. In the winter, all exercises should be adapted for cross-country skis so that they may be worn at all times.

Because of the skis, try not to cross many roads. The road surface may damage the skis, requiring their removal. Second, skiers may have trouble mounting snow banks at the road edges.

Curves in the fitness trail should be smooth rather than sharp to facilitate use by cross-country skiers in the winter.

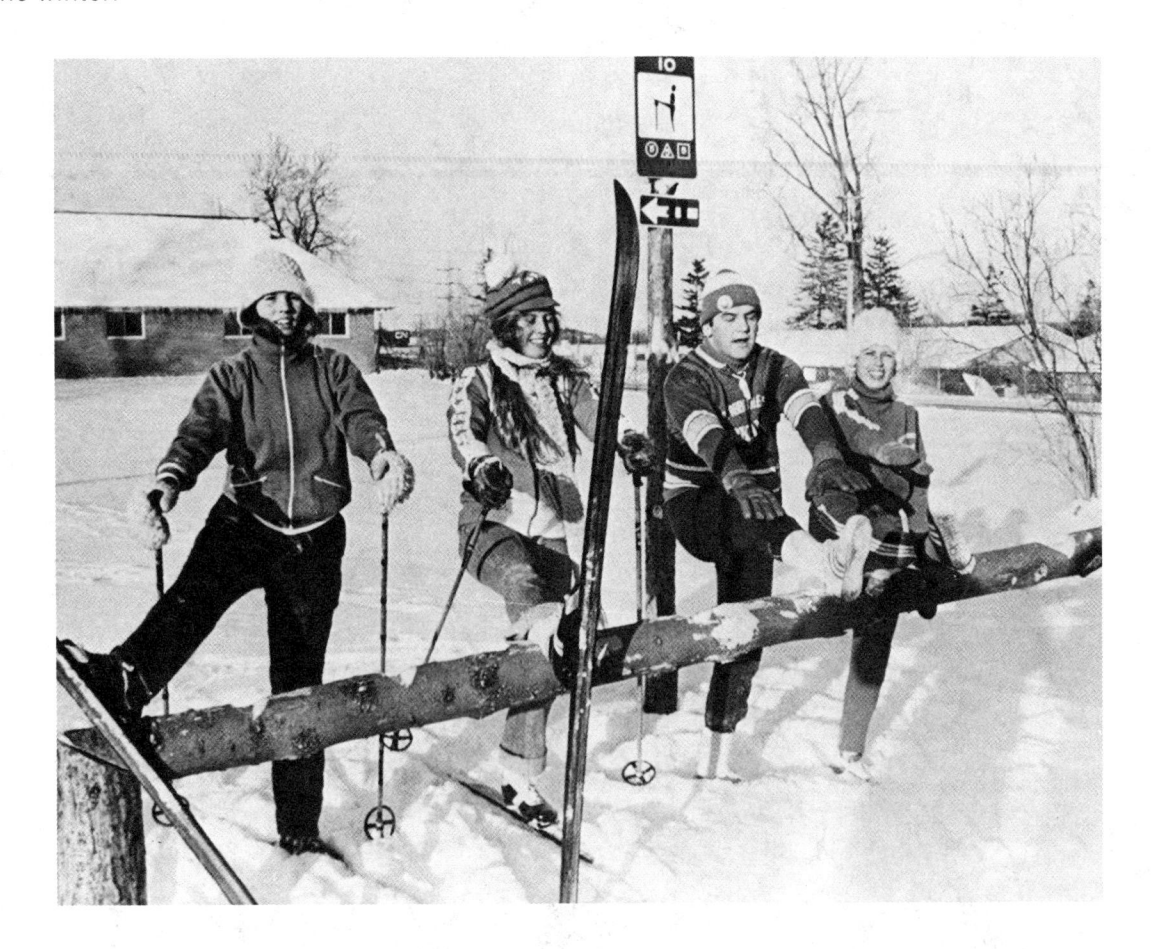

FITNESS TRAIL SITE SELECTION

Where you locate your fitness trail is a key factor in its ultimate use. Whether in an urban or rural setting, certain guidelines will more likely ensure success.

1. Select a piece of land which will permit a 1- to 2-minute jogging circuit with 10 to 20 exercise stations.
2. It should be easily accessible to people.
3. If possible, select land that is already used by people, therefore ensuring a ready-made population to use the fitness trail.
4. It would be helpful if the land surrounding the site is also well established for use, e.g., playing fields or picnic areas. Therefore the fitness trail can be used as a warm-up before a practice in a sport, e.g., football, baseball, soccer, etc. Or, as fitness is a family affair, the fun aspect can be encouraged by family picnics mixed with physical activity. The ultimate aim of encouraging more people to get fit through involvement in physical activity will also be promoted as they have the opportunity to participate and use other recreational facilities such as a swimming pool; tennis, volleyball, badminton, squash, or handball courts; or gym facilities.
5. Take advantage of what you have: land with lots of trees, interesting contours, elevations, natural vegetation, open spaces.
6. Do not select delicate ecological areas which can be easily damaged when used by great numbers of people.
7. Natural vegetation will beautify the fitness trail and will also partially screen it from view. This is desirable for those who are shy.
8. The beginning and the end of the trail should be in the same area. A parking lot should be close to the start; showers and a water fountain near the end. By using existing recreational facilities, these may already be available and will thus reduce the overall cost of this fitness project.
9. Place park benches throughout the trail for people to rest on. This might be of particular benefit for senior citizens and young children.
10. Changes in elevation should not occur at the beginning of the fitness trail as they may prove to be too strenuous for some participants and discourage them from using the trail.
11. Make sure you have written permission to use the site you choose, if necessary.

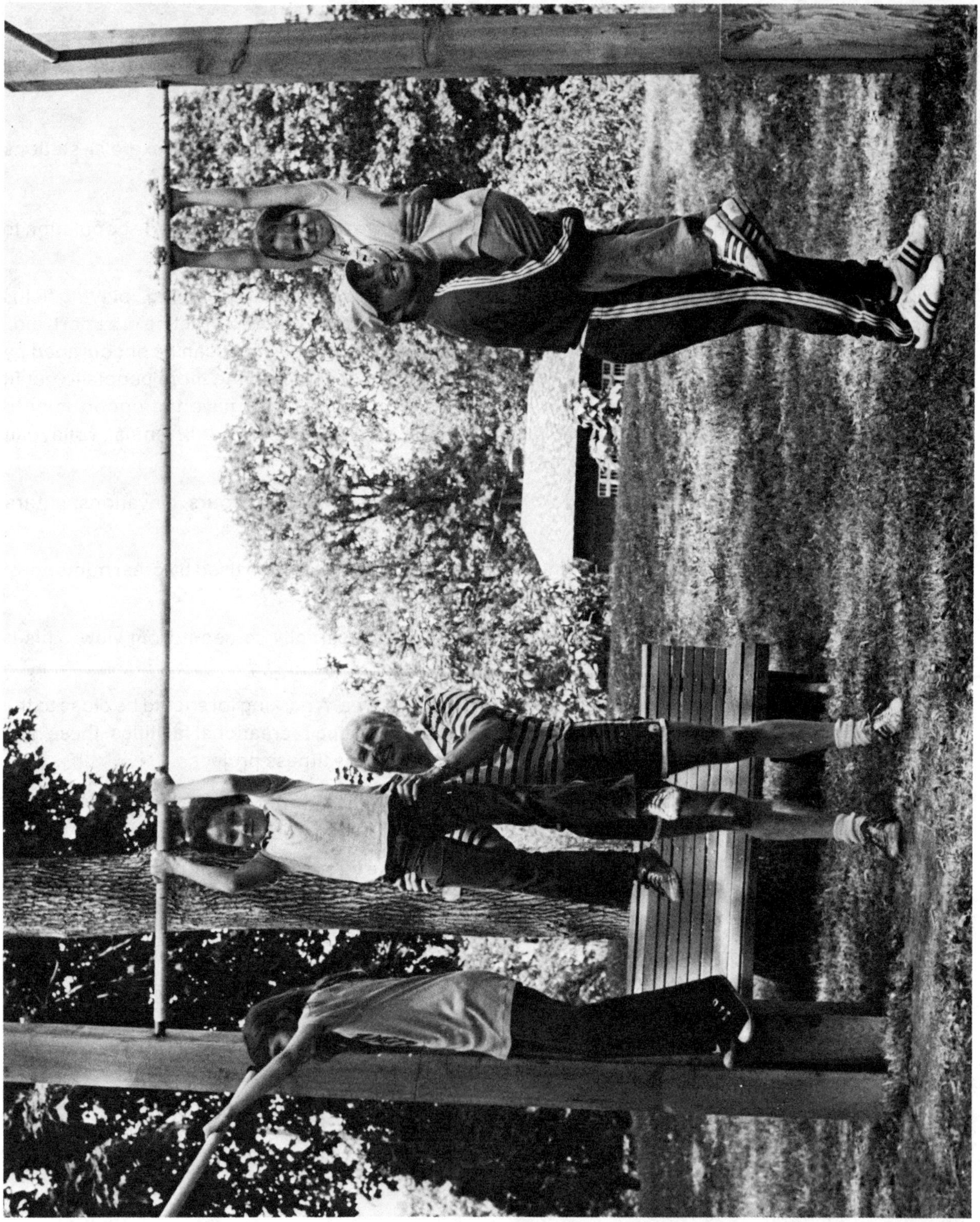

SELECTION AND DESIGN OF FITNESS TRAIL EQUIPMENT

One way to reduce accident risk is to use great care in selection and construction of fitness trail equipment. Also, the fewer pieces of apparatus, the cheaper and easier it is to build a fitness trail.

These tips might help you with the fitness trail equipment you do decide to install.

1. Mix apparatus and nonapparatus stations throughout the trail.
2. All apparatus should be permanent: posts sunk 3 feet into the ground and cemented there.
3. Apparatus should be adaptable to all ages and heights and sex of the participants, e.g., slant bars or provide two or three heights.
4. Several people of different or similar builds should be able to use the apparatus simultaneously.
5. Apparatus is most cheaply built using telephone and hydro poles, and railway ties to achieve a rustic look for the fitness trail.
6. All apparatus should be treated with wood preservatives to arrest deterioration.
7. All rough edges should be smoothed carefully.
8. All nails, spikes, bolts, etc. used to build the apparatus should be recessed so that no one will be injured.
9. Don't include any apparatus that needs constant care.
10. The injury rate on certain pieces of fitness trail equipment apparatus may prove that the exercises are of less benefit and more risk. For instance, one exercise requires participants to leap frog over posts, of increasing height, embedded in cement. See Figure 9. Very dangerous. Another exercise which could badly damage the knees is the hurdle jump. See Figure 10. Since the hurdles will not tip over if you hit them, guess what has to give instead? Certain exercises put undue stress on vulnerable joints such as the knees and muscles of the body, e.g., the back (see Figure 11). In designing fitness trails apparatus, it is important not to include exercises where participants could easily slip, fall, and strike their bodies, particularly their head. Two that are very dangerous, yet seen often, are jumping from log top to log top (see Figure 12), and jumping from side to side over a log (see Figure 13).

Some fitness apparatus is also impractical; for instance those that use sand. People steal it to make cement, kids play in it, it is washed away by rain, etc. One popular European exercise is to lift logs of varying weights, (see Figure 14). People can steal these logs for firewood unless they are securely fastened. Don't incorporate any apparatus where parts of it are easily taken, such as ropes or rings, or you will constantly be maintaining and repairing your fitness trail (see Figures 15 and 16).

Equipment To Avoid

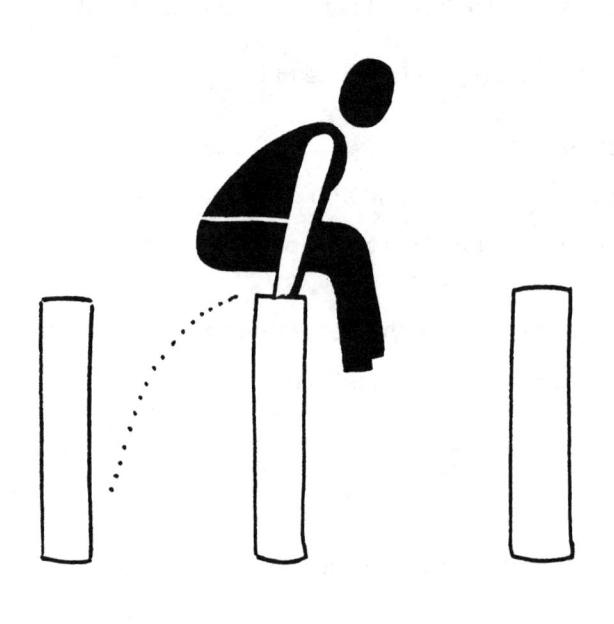

Figure 9

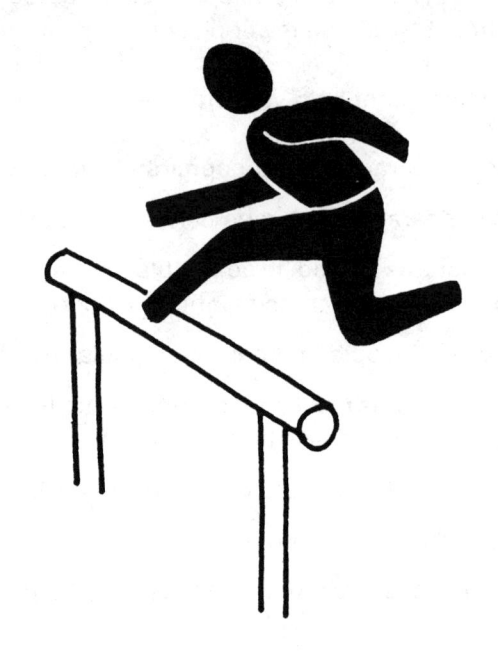

Figure 10

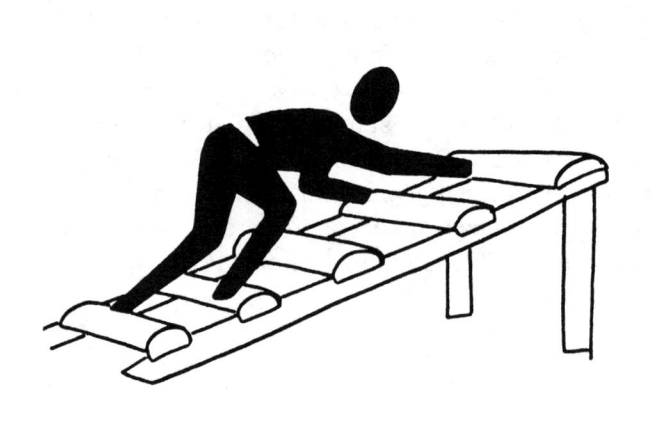

Figure 11

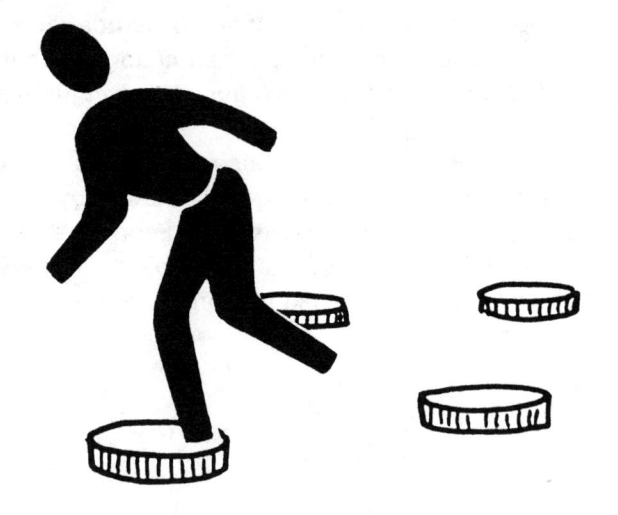

Figure 12

Equipment To Avoid

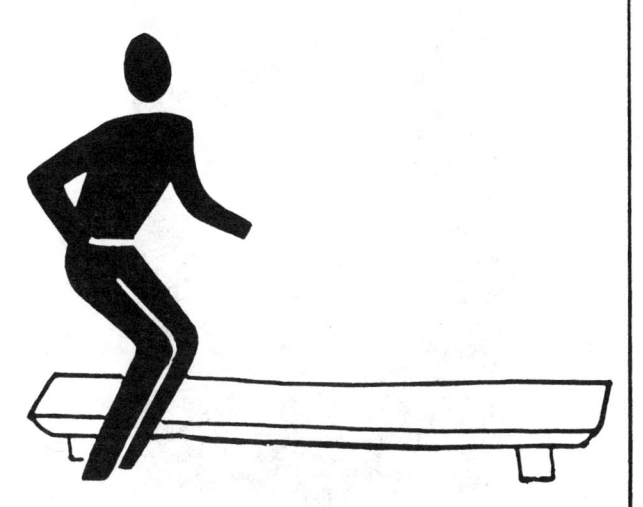

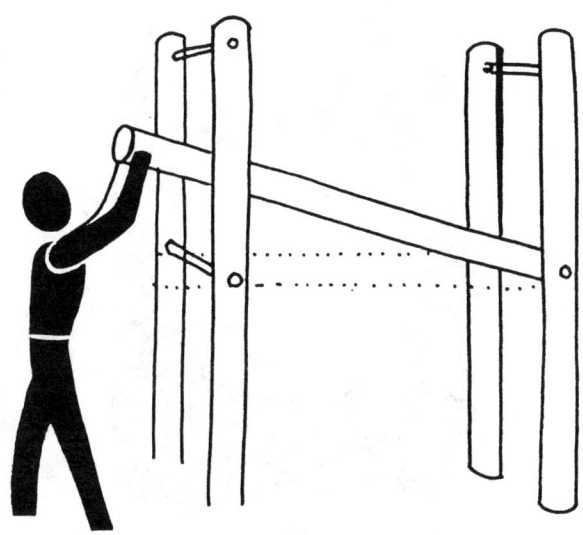

Figure 13

Figure 14

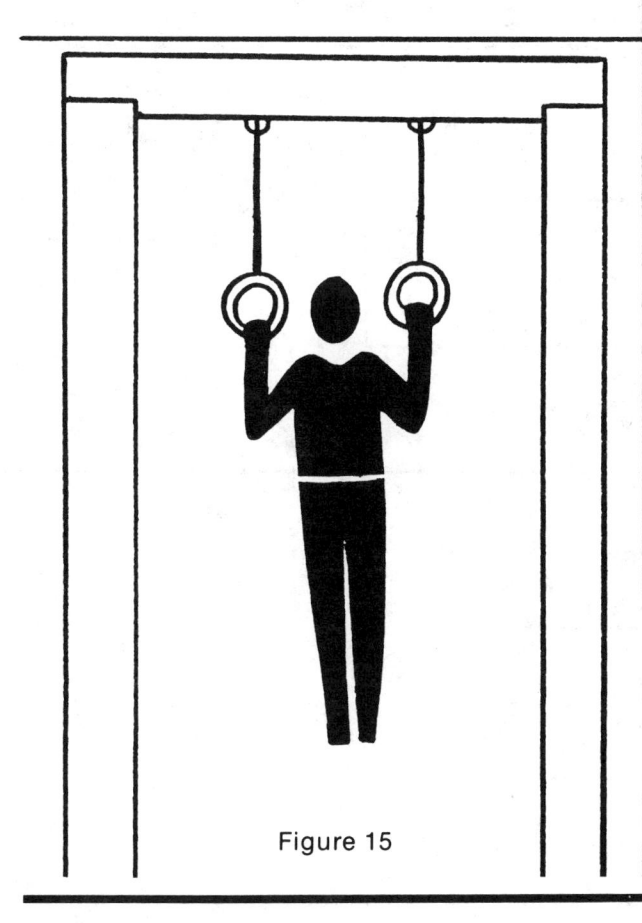

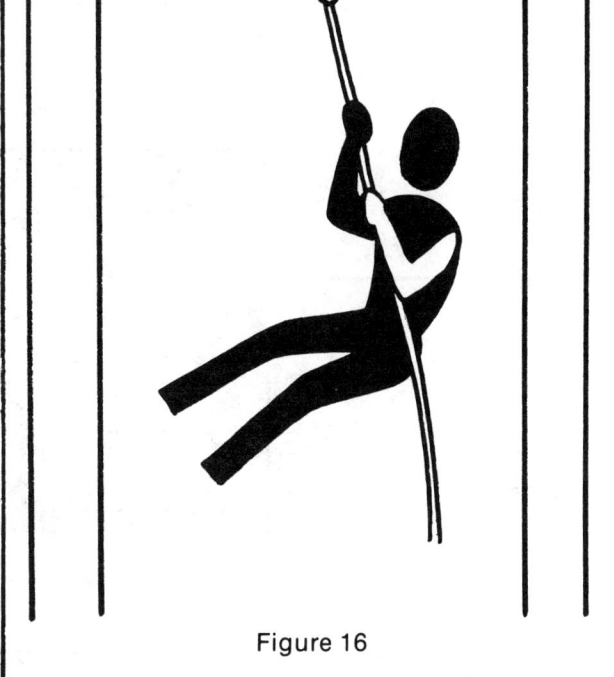

Figure 15

Figure 16

Some Sample Signs

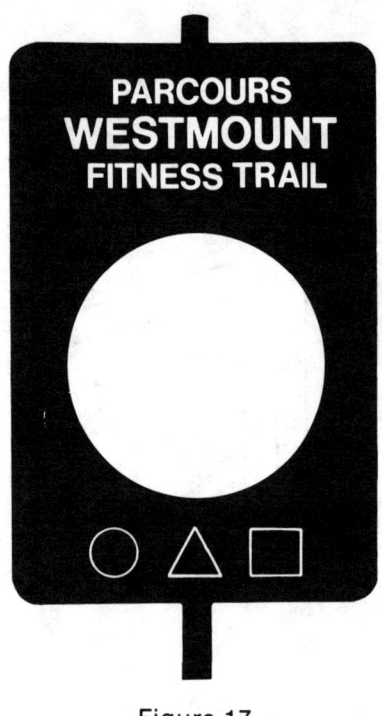

Figure 17

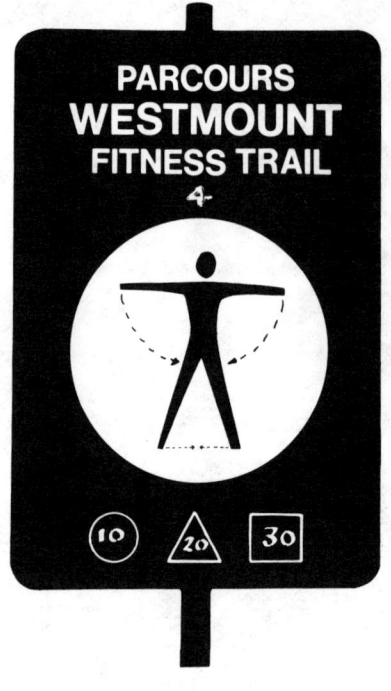

Figure 18

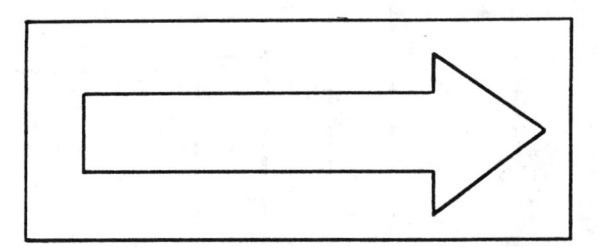

Figure 19

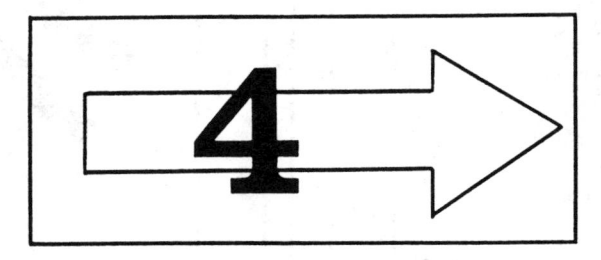

Figure 20

FITNESS TRAIL SIGNS

Signs will most likely be your largest expense in setting up a fitness trail. Here are some tips which will reduce this expense.

1. Have your artwork done locally. If you are part of a school or city recreation department, they may have their own graphic artists or get better deals with certain local ones.
2. Get together with another organization or organizations that are interested in constructing a fitness trail and mass produce your signs.
3. Mass print your main signs, i.e., exercise plaques and directional arrows. It's cheaper. You can fill in the details later, such as pictures of exercises, number of repetitions, station numbers. See Figures 17 and 18.
4. Pictures on signs should be nonsexist to eliminate any confusion or criticism (see below).

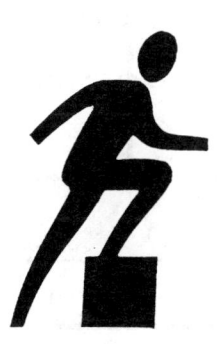

5. Signs should contain few words as the sign will increase in cost per unit. Your introductory sign is the notable exception.
6. Preferably, signs should be made of metal. Use galvanized steel made for the outdoors –032 aluminum. Wood signs can be vandalized more easily, e.g., carved or shot up with BB guns. Wood also rots eventually.
7. Metal signs can be backed with wood to increase their durability.
8. Usually red, black, or blue on white are the cheapest colors to have on your signs. School colors could be used but unless they are of the above combinations, they are likely to be more expensive. Make sure your color choices stick out, i.e., they don't blend into the background trees, etc. Blue tends to do this.
9. Try florescent paint if it's not too costly and suits your purposes.
10. When you have your main signs printed (exercise plaques and directional arrows), run off extra blanks so you can replace signs quickly when needed. Also, the more signs you have printed, the cheaper each one becomes.
11. Directional arrows should be separate from the main exercise plaques in case you decide to change the placement of a station and the arrow indicating the direction of the next station now points in the wrong direction. See Figure 19.
12. If you wish to number the directional arrows, indicating what station lies ahead, and where, paint on the numbers yourself. Buy a large set of stencils specifically for this purpose; trace the number on in pen, then paint it in a color that stands out. See Figure 20.

SIGNS REQUIRED

The quantity of each sign will depend on the design of your particular fitness trail.

a. "Start" sign	START / DEBUT	10" X 14" 032 aluminum
b. "Finish" sign	END / FIN	8" X 8" 032 aluminum
c. "Short circuit" signs	SHORT CIRCUIT FOR 1 MILE COURSE / CIRCUIT RACCOURCI 1 MILLE	12" X 18" 032 aluminum
d. "End of Short Circuit" sign	END OF SHORT CIRCUIT / FIN DE CIRCUIT RACCOURCI	10" X 12" 032 aluminum
e. "And/Or" signs	and/or / l'un ou l'autre	5" X 12" 032 aluminum

f. "Winter signs"	WINTER / HIVER	5" X 24" 032 aluminum
g. Exercise station signs	PARCOURS WESTMOUNT FITNESS TRAIL	12" X 24" 032 aluminum
h. Arrows	→	12" X 5" 032 aluminum
i. Introductory instruction sign	Parcours Westmount Fitness Trail / French / English	4' X 5' 020 aluminum (sign backed in ½ inch plywood)

49

Figure 21

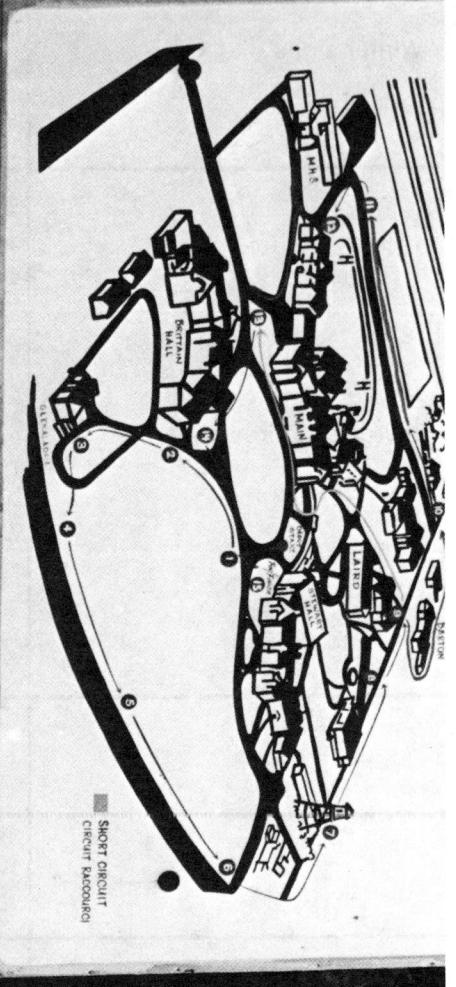

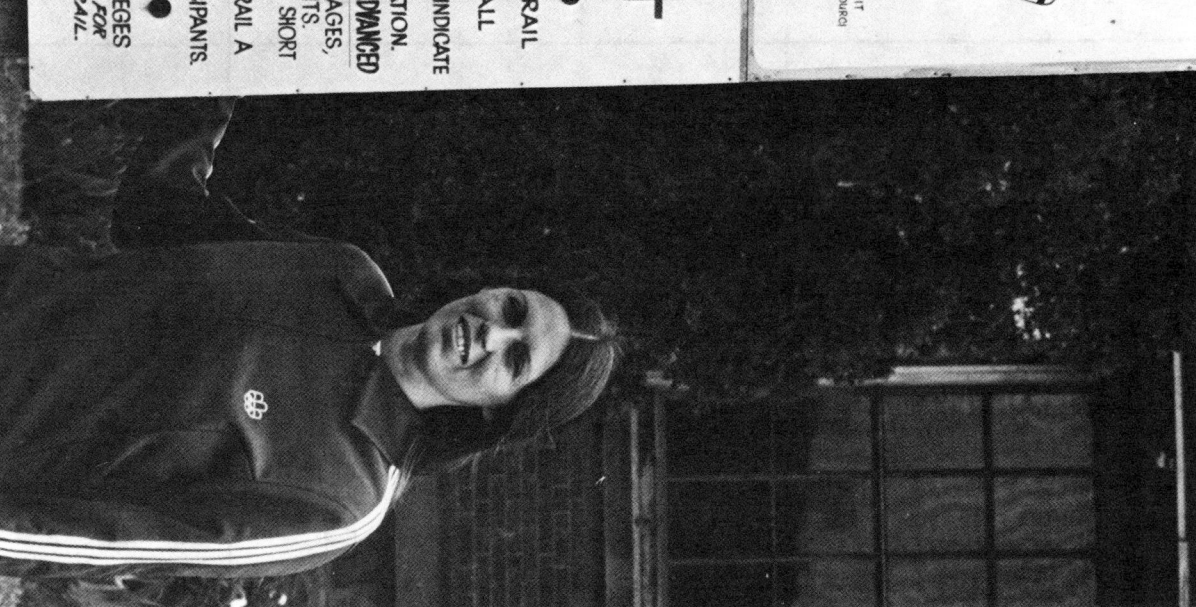

PURPOSES OF THE SIGNS

a. and b. **Start and Finish signs**—required to clearly indicate the beginning and the end of the trail.

c. and d. **Short Circuit signs and Short Circuit Ends signs**—required to clearly indicate the pathway of the short circuit trail.

e. **And/Or signs**—required at stations where more than one exercise can be performed on the same piece of equipment—to be used in between the two exercise plaques, e.g., chin-ups or body circles could both be done on the chin-up bar. Put signs up for both exercises for the benefit of regular users of the trail, giving them a choice of exercises, eliminating boredom caused by constant repetition of the same exercises.

f. **Winter signs**—may be used to indicate exercises which should be done only in the winter on cross-country skis. If you use these signs, you will never have to change exercise plaques—as you must otherwise do twice a year (spring and fall) to adjust for the seasonal changes in exercises.

g. **Exercise plaques**—required to indicate the station number, the exercise to be performed, and the suggested repetitions to be performed by each level of participant—beginner, intermediate, and advanced (using a circle, a triangle, and a square).

   e.g.,   ◯ BEGINNER   ☐ INTERMEDIATE   △ ADVANCED

h. **Directional arrows**—required at the bottom of each exercise plaque to indicate the direction of the next exercise station. They are also used to clearly indicate any changes in direction that may occur between stations, removing any doubt as to the direction to be taken.

i. **Introductory sign**—to explain:
   - How to use the fitness trail.
   - Who paid for the trail (optional).
   - Who designed the trail (optional).
   - How often to use the trail.
   - A medical checkup is suggested.
   - May include a liability clause, i.e., that the organization who constructed the fitness trail is not responsible for accidents, etc. occurring on it.
   - To explain the short circuit (if there is one).
   - A map of the fitness trail to show the location of the exercise stations.
   - How long the trail is.
   - How many exercise stations are included.
   - Location of washrooms, telephones, showers, locker rooms (optional).
   - Hours of use (optional).

   Place the introductory sign in a place that is clearly visible, close to the start of the fitness trail, to draw attention to it.

Figure 22

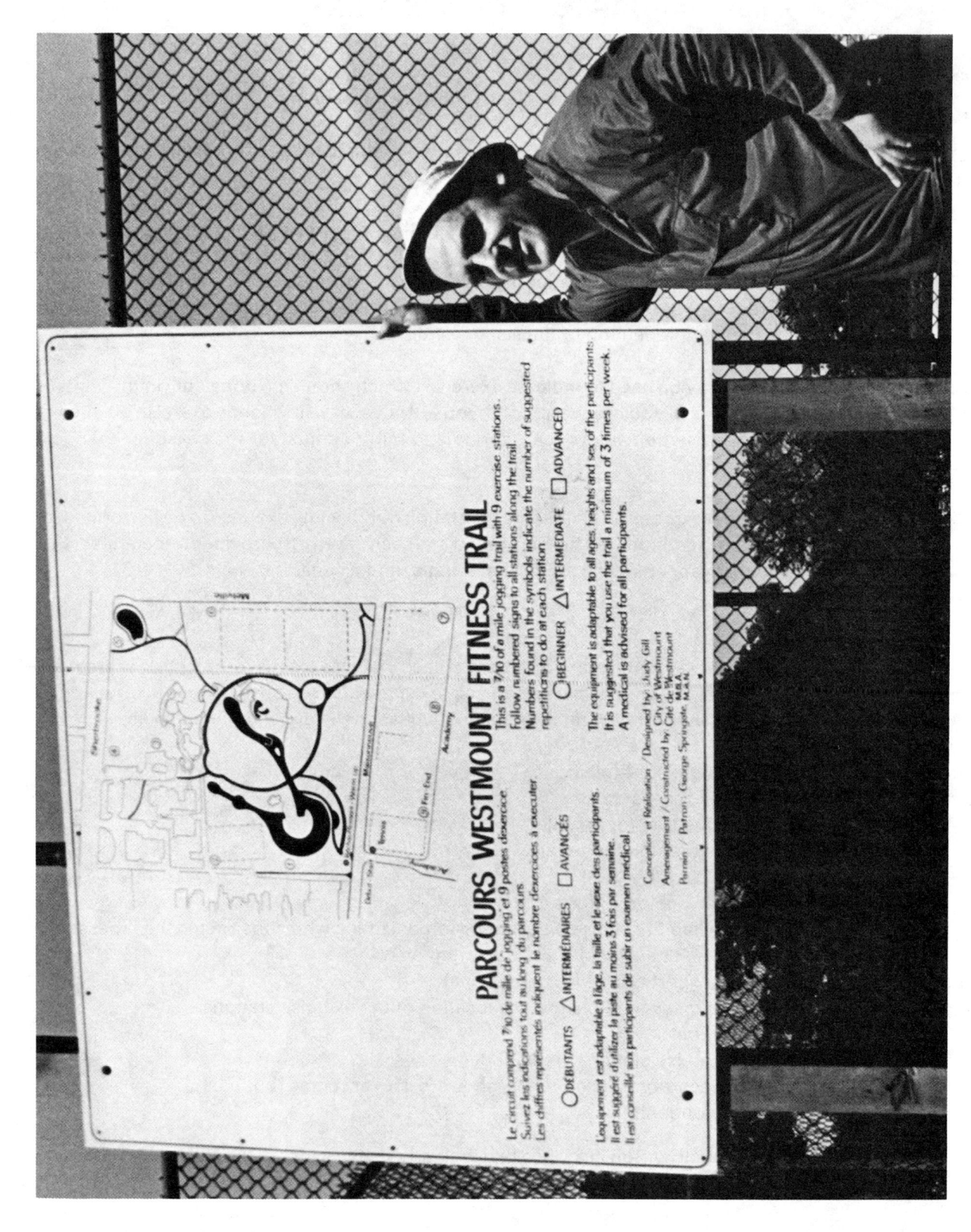

BILINGUAL SIGNS

If there is a second language (French, Spanish, etc.) used frequently by potential users of the fitness trail, consider making your trail bilingual.

a. EXAMPLE: a bilingual exercise plaque—see below.

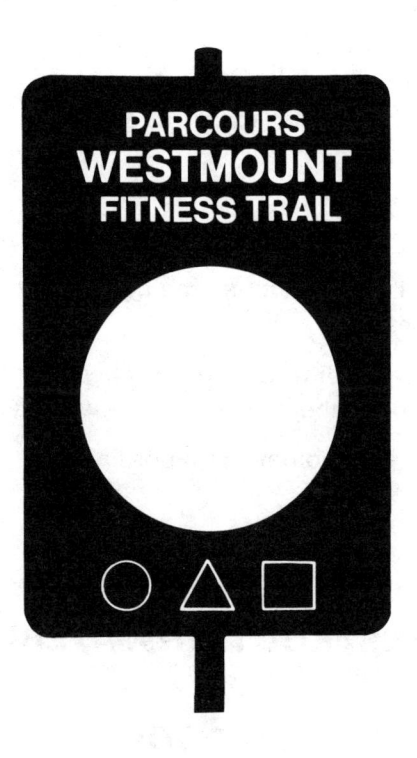

b. EXAMPLE: a bilingual introductory sign—see Figures 21 and 22.

FITNESS TRAIL CONSTRUCTION PREPARATIONS

1. Buy all required materials at one time—wood, hardware, equipment.

2. Prepare wood
   a. Preserve wood.
   b. Drill holes for bolting in signs.

3. Prepare signs
   a. Drill signs to be bolted onto signposts.
   b. Paint in station numbers on directional arrows if required.

4. Prepare trail site
   a. Dig all holes required.

5. Prepare cement
   a. Obtain tools and equipment required to lay the cement, e.g., water bucket, water, water hose, mixing pallette, shovels, hoe.

6. Arrange for transportation—a truck or tractor to carry people, building materials (signs, signposts, other wood) and equipment around the fitness trail site while constructing it.

7. Arrange for people to build the trail, volunteers if possible.

CONSTRUCTION MATERIALS

WOOD:

The quantity of wood required to build a fitness trail will vary greatly according to how long your trail is, how many exercise stations you have, and how much equipment is required at each. Telephone or hydro poles and railway ties can be used for this purpose. Trees from a neighborhood arboretum may sometimes be obtained at low cost when purchased in bulk.

It is very important to preserve all wood used to build apparatus, signposts, etc. with wood preservatives.

Certain wood requirements can be predicted:

List: One-12 foot post at each exercise station.
Signposts for short circuit trail.
Signpost for the introductory sign.
Signposts for start and finish signs.
Signposts for directional arrows that are not attached to exercise plaque posts. These are used to clarify the direction to be taken when there is a choice of pathways, e.g., in an open field, in a thick forest, etc.
Wood for each exercise station that uses equipment.

TOOLS AND EQUIPMENT:

Borrow as much as possible. Rent the rest as required.

List:
- Truck or tractor
- Chainsaw, with oil and gas
- Stepladders
- Electric drill, with wood and metal bits
- Axes
- Wrenches
- Hammers
- Tape measures
- Paint brushes
- Gas-run post hole digger—2-man or tractor operated
- Auger—8 to 10 inch
- Line bars
- Shovels
- Split shovels—to dig dirt out of holes
- Buckets
- Water hose
- Cement mixing unit

MATERIALS:

The materials to construct your fitness trail depend a great deal on the design and choice of exercises to be used at the exercise stations. The following is a partial list of what might be required.

List:
- Wood
- Wood preservative
- Bolts
- Washers
- Spikes—10 inch
- Brackets—for Chin-Up Bar Station
- Metal bars—4 for Chin-Up Bar Station
- Tape—to wrap around the chin-up bars so wet hands won't stick to them in the winter
- Door numbers—for Sergeant's Jump station
- Cement
- Oil and gas—for chainsaw
- Sign paint—for directional arrows to apply numbers and touch-ups as required
- Brushes, paint cleaner, containers for touch-up paint
- Stencils—4 inch for directional arrows
- Pamphlet box—for instruction booklets on how to use the fitness trail

LABOR

Try to enlist as much volunteer help as possible as this will significantly reduce the cost of constructing your fitness trail. Local community organizations; boys'/girls' and men's/women's clubs; schools, colleges, and universities (forestry, physical education, and recreation departments) are all potential sources of aid.

Other Considerations in Construction of a Fitness Trail

1. Touch-up sign paint is needed for application of numbers to directional arrows and to use for repairs.

2. Premixed cement, although more expensive than regular dry cement mix, is easier and much faster to use, and requires less help.

3. Foot surface: Wood chips are quite commonly used as foot surfacing to soften the impact when the foot hits the ground while running. However, wood chips are quite expensive requiring specialized equipment to make them and a ready source of wood. The chips tend to scatter off pathways as well thus demanding constant maintenance to keep them in place. For the expense and maintenance problems, grass or dirt tracks might do as well.

4. Lighting: This is an added attraction to your fitness trail if you can afford it. It promotes safety of participants and night time use of the trail.

INSURANCE

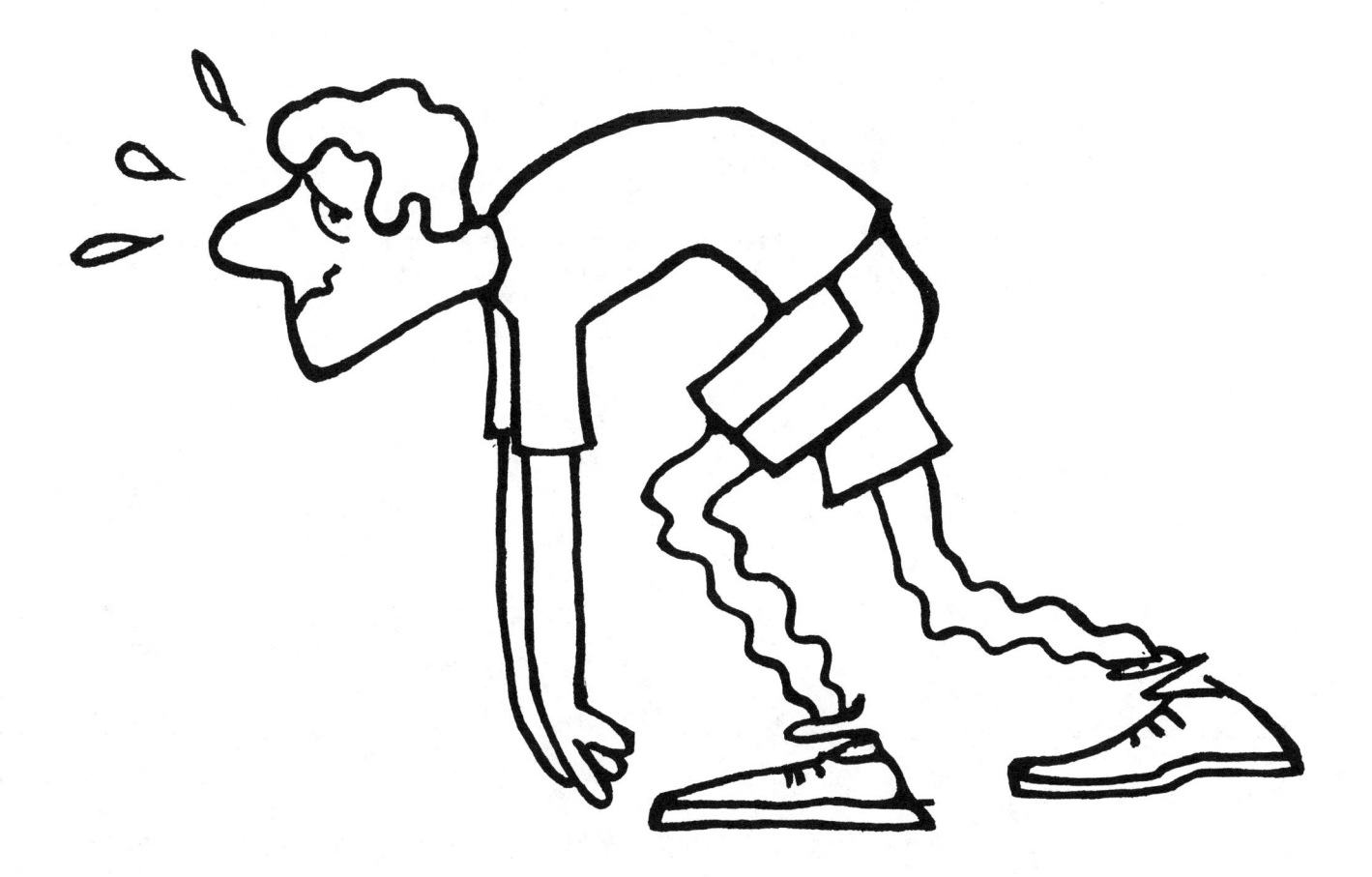

Obtain insurance for the fitness trail. If it is incorporated into existing recreational facilities, it is possible that an umbrella policy already exists which can be extended to include the trail as well. Adequate public liability is an absolute necessity to cover all eventualities. Check with an insurance company for more details.

SAMPLE BUDGET FOR A FITNESS TRAIL

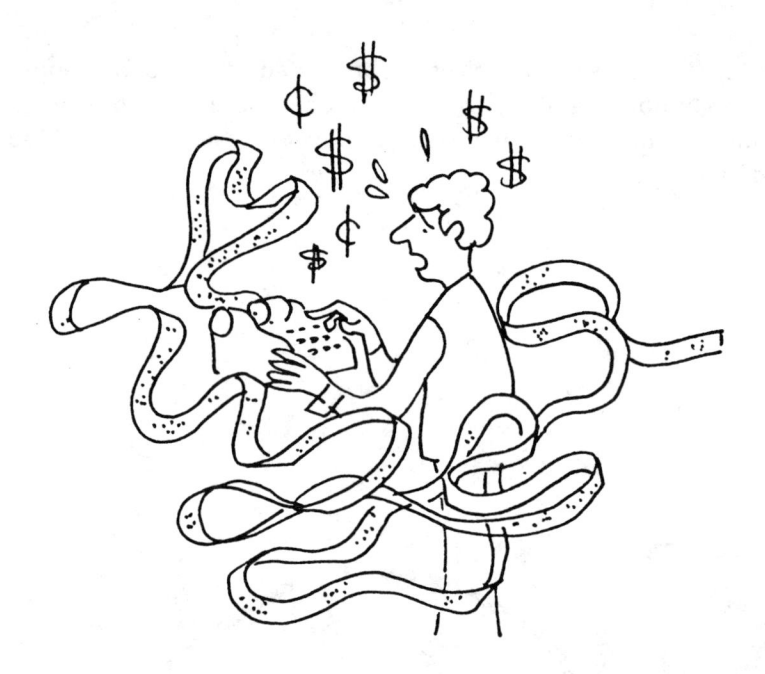

Much depends on what you are able to obtain for free. Note: These are approximate costs. Prices will also vary according to the part of the country in which the trail is constructed.

SIGNS

Signs	$3,000.00	
Artwork	300.00	
Extra signs	350.00	
	$3,650.00	$3,650.00

PRINTING

Pamphlets	$ 300.00	$ 300.00

PUBLICITY

Slides, film, prints	$ 200.00	$ 200.00

EQUIPMENT RENTAL

Tools, etc.	$ 300.00	$ 300.00

BUILDING MATERIALS

Wood, hardware, etc.	$ 500.00	$ 500.00

LABOR

	?	?
		$4,950.00

CONSTRUCTION DETAILS

A cleared-out nook is needed for each exercise station, to the side of the jogging circuit, so as not to impede other participants. Sign posts are needed at each station.

NO EQUIPMENT NEEDED
exercises k-t (excluding q)

EACH STATION
Wood:
1 X 12' log — 5" diameter

Hardware & Supplies:
3 bolts
3 washers

Holes:
1

Signs:
1 exercise sign
1 arrow

SIGN POST
12-foot posts are suggested (cedar are the best), sunk 3 feet into the ground (below the frost line so the cement won't heave), and fixed in with cement to prevent vandalism and to make the installations permanent. The signs are placed 9 feet above the ground to prevent damage.

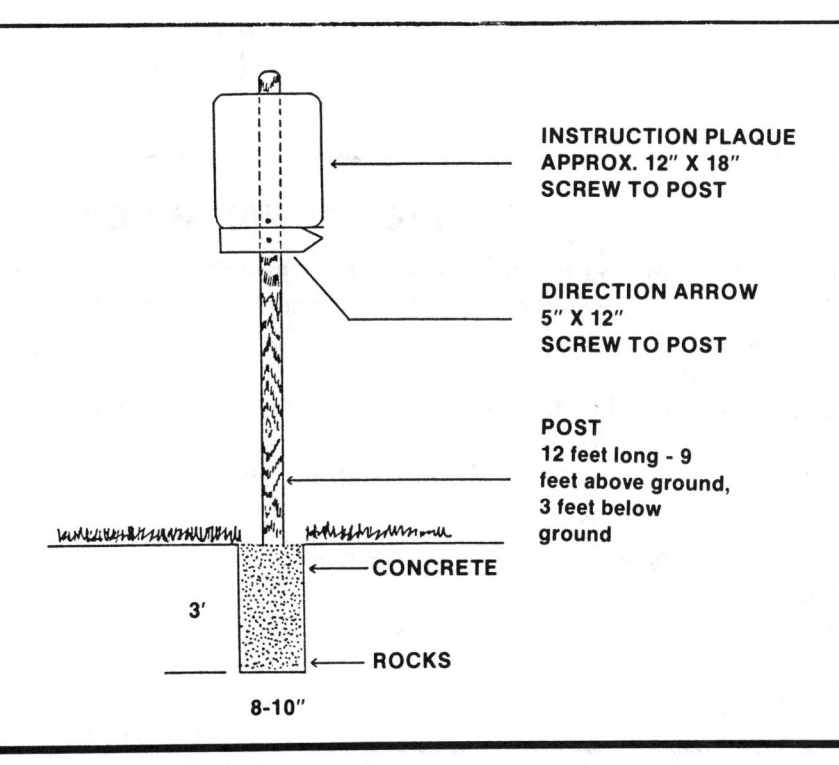

Construction Details:

- INSTRUCTION PLAQUE APPROX. 12" X 18" SCREW TO POST
- DIRECTION ARROW 5" X 12" SCREW TO POST
- POST 12 feet long - 9 feet above ground, 3 feet below ground
- CONCRETE
- 3'
- ROCKS
- 8-10"

SHORT CIRCUIT SIGNS

The following is required for each short circuit that is installed:

Wood:
1 X 12' log—5" diameter

Holes:
1

Hardware & Supplies:
3 bolts
3 washers

Signs:
1 short circuit sign
　　　or
1 short circuit ends sign
1 directional arrow (if use "short circuit" sign)

Construction Details:
Same as exercise stations where no equipment is required.

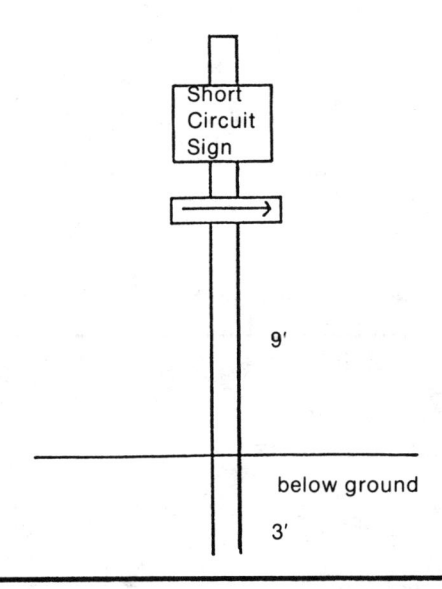

```
    ┌──────┐
    │Short │
    │Circuit│
    │Sign  │
    └──────┘
    ┌──→───┐
    └──────┘
           │
           │ 9'
           │
    ───────┼───────
           │ below ground
           │ 3'
```

DIRECTIONAL ARROWS

Most directional arrows are attached below exercise station plaques. However, there are times when a path may divide into two or more and there is some question as to which direction must be taken. A directional arrow would be located here.

The following is required for each directional arrow that is installed:

Wood:
1 X 12' log — 5" diameter

Hardware & Supplies
1 bolt
1 washer

Holes:
1

Signs:
1 directional arrow

Construction Details:
Same as above.

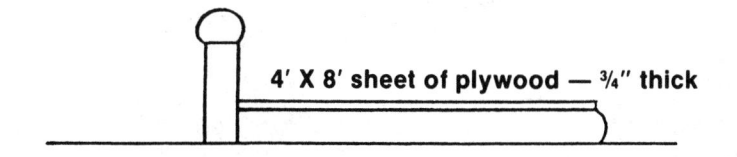

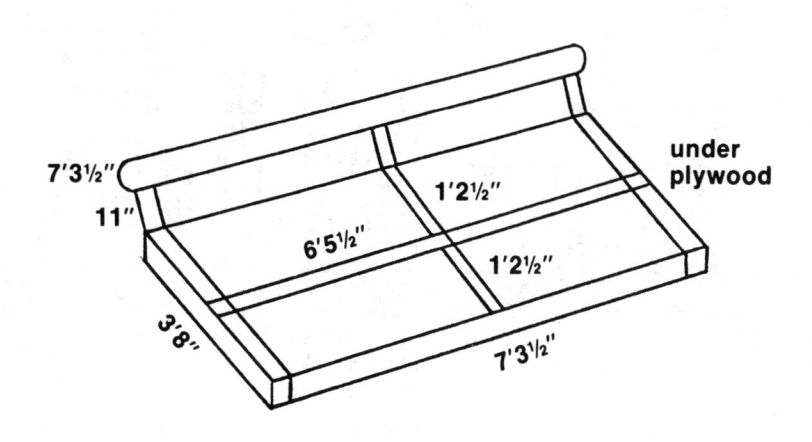

SIT-UPS AND CHEST RAISES

Wood:
1 X 12' log — 5" diameter
3 X 7'3½" logs — 5" diameter
3 X 11" logs — 5" diameter
2 X 3'8" logs — 5" diameter
2 X 1'2½" logs — 5" diameter
1 X 6'5½" log — 5" diameter
1 piece of ¾" plywood — 4' X 8'

Hardware & Supplies:

Winter	Summer	
3 bolts	6 bolts	1 paint brush
3 washers	6 washers	15 finishing nails - 3" long
	12 spikes — 10" long	1 quart of clear pentox

Holes:
1

Signs:

Winter	Summer
1 exercise sign	2 exercise signs
1 arrow	1 arrow
	1 and/or sign

Construction Details:

4' X 8' sheet of plywood — ¾" thick

7'3½"
11"
6'5½"
1'2½"
1'2½"
3'8"
7'3½"
under plywood

STEP-UPS

Wood:
1 X 12' log — 5" diameter
5 logs of misc. heights & widths for e.g.
   1 X 15" log — 1'10" diameter
   1 X 1'7½" log — 1'7" diameter
   1 X 10" log — 2' diameter
   + 2 others

Hardware & Supplies:
3 bolts
3 washers

Holes:
1

Signs:
1 exercise sign
1 arrow

Construction Details:

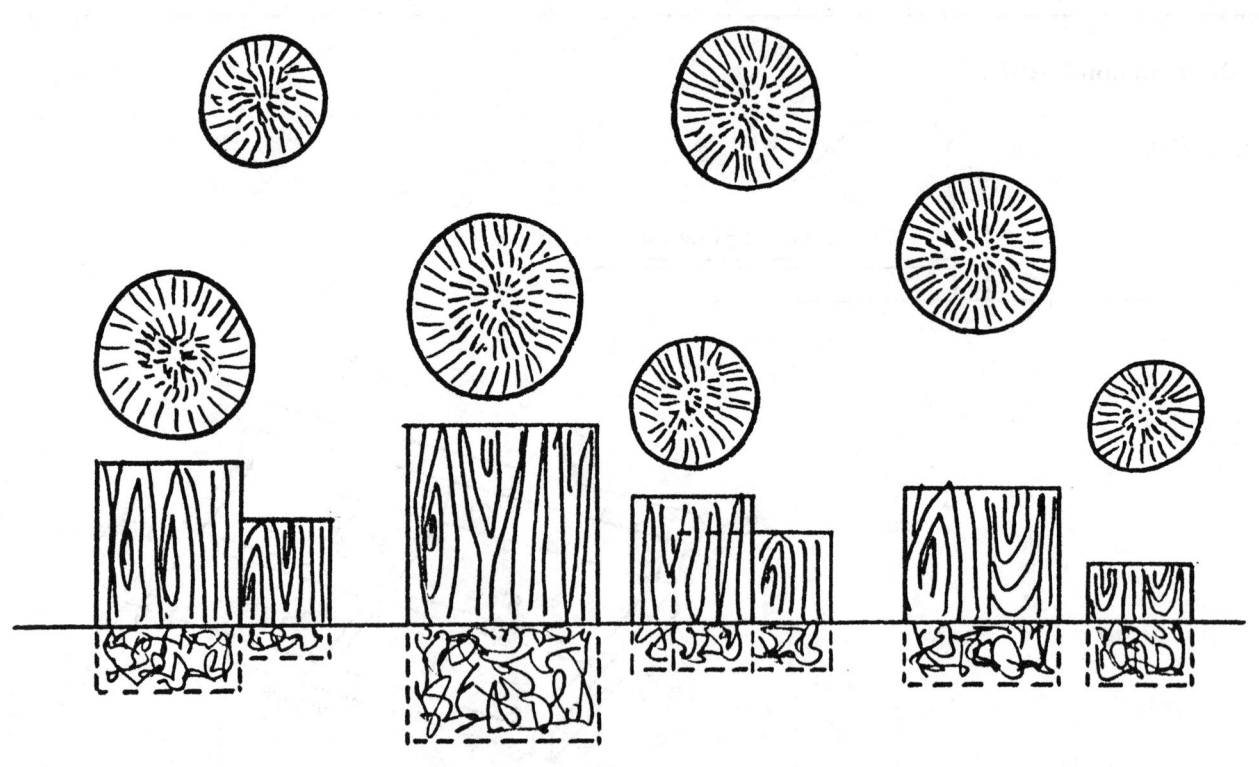

(use assorted tree stumps and trunks, — 12"-24" dia. and 12"-24" high scattered irregularly)

HURDLER'S DRILL

Wood:
1 X 12' log — 5" diameter
1 X 4'7" log — 5" diameter
1 X 6'2" log — 5" diameter
1 X 12'2" log — 5" diameter

Hardware & Supplies:
3 bolts
3 washers
3 spikes — 10" long

Holes:
3

Signs:
1 exercise sign
1 arrow

Special Instructions:
— cut heel cups with a chainsaw every foot

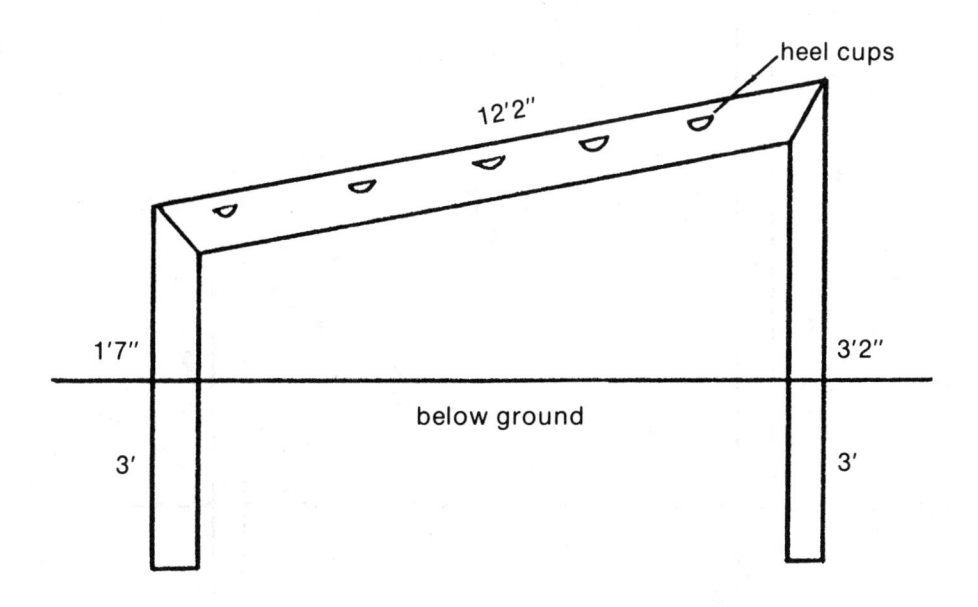

Construction Details:

63

SERGEANT'S JUMP

Wood:
1 X 12' log — 5" diameter
1 X 11'10" log — 5" diameter
1 X 10'1" log — 5" diameter
1 X 8'6" log — diameter

Hardware & Supplies:
3 bolts
3 washers
2 spikes — 10" long
Door Numbers — 5, 6, 7, 8

Holes:
3

Signs:
1 exercise sign
1 arrow

Construction Details:

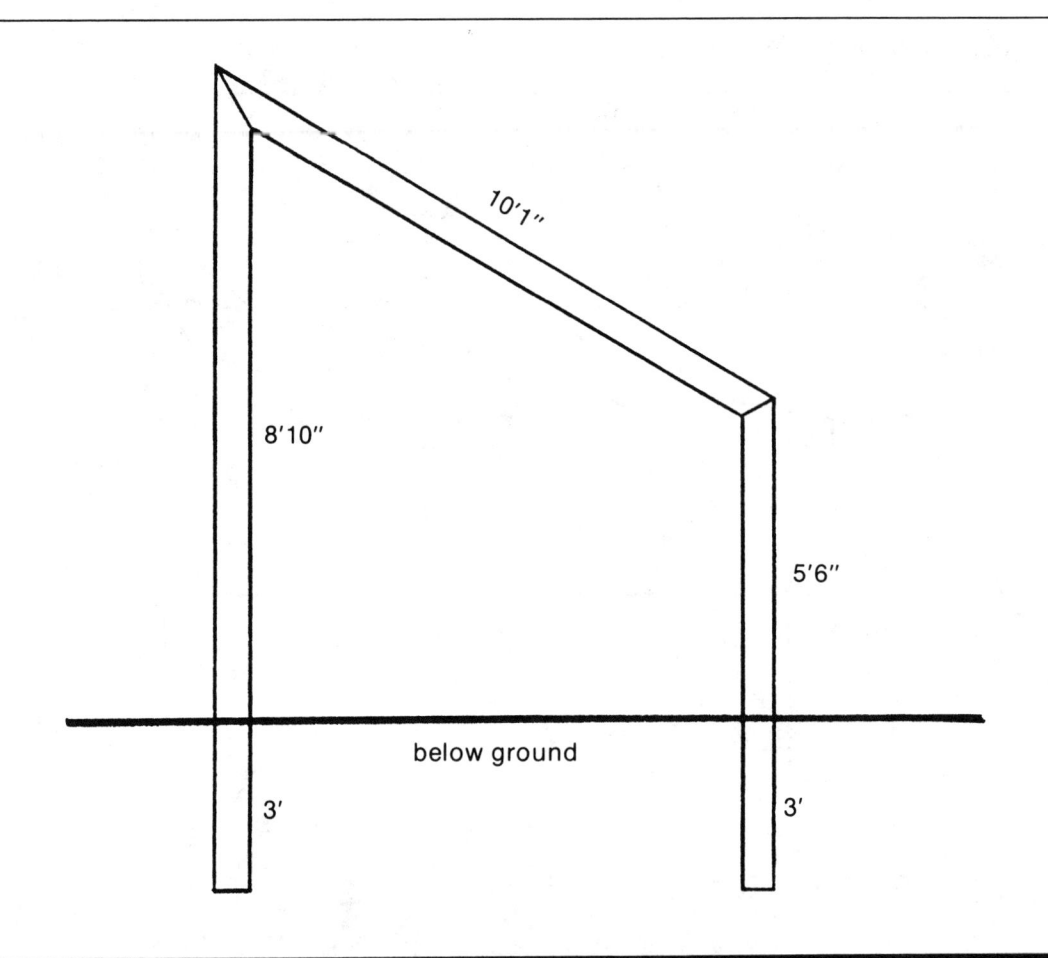

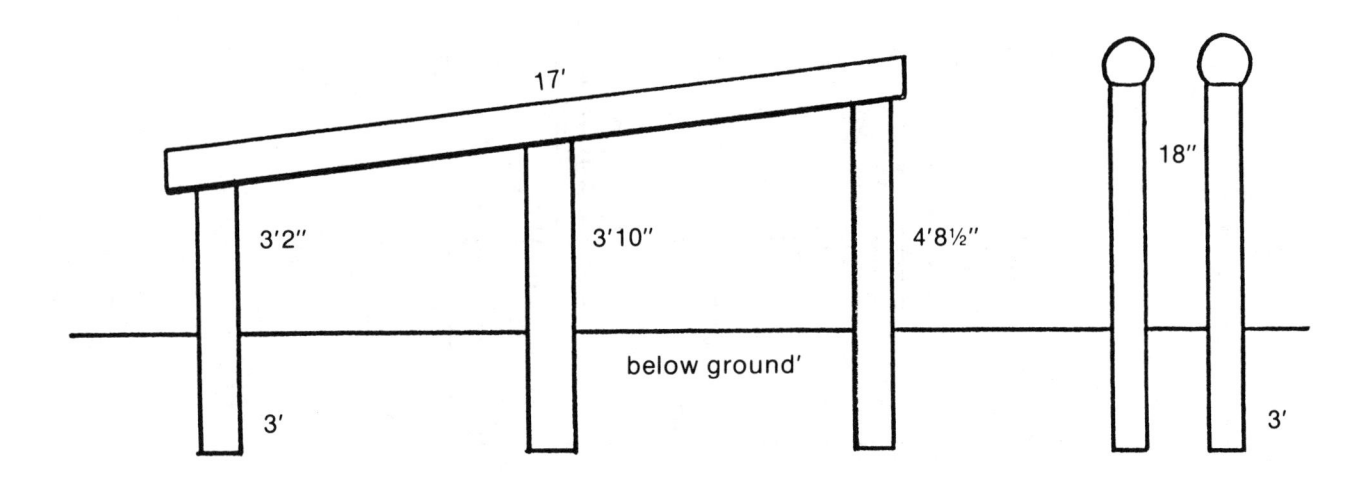

HANDWALK AND DIPS

Wood:
1 X 12' log — 5" diameter
2 X 17' logs — 5" diameter
2 X 5'2" logs — 5" diameter
2 X 6'10" logs — diameter
2 X 7'8½" logs — 5" diameter

Hardware & Supplies:
6 bolts
6 washers
6 spikes — 10" long

Holes:
7

Signs:

Winter	Summer
1 exercise sign	2 exercise signs
1 arrow	1 arrow
	1 and/or sign

Construction Details:

BODY CIRCLES AND CHIN-UPS

Wood:
5 X 12' logs — 5" diameter
1 X 4'5" log — 5" diameter
1 X 3'6½" log — 5" diameter
1 X 4'2" log — 5" diameter
1 X 5'½" log — 5" diameter

Hardware & Supplies:
6 bolts
6 washers
16 spikes — 10" long
16 brackets
9½ rolls of tape - 20' long 1½" wide
4 metal bars - 9' long, ¼" diameter

Holes:
9

Signs:
2 exercise signs
1 arrow
1 and/or sign

Construction Details:

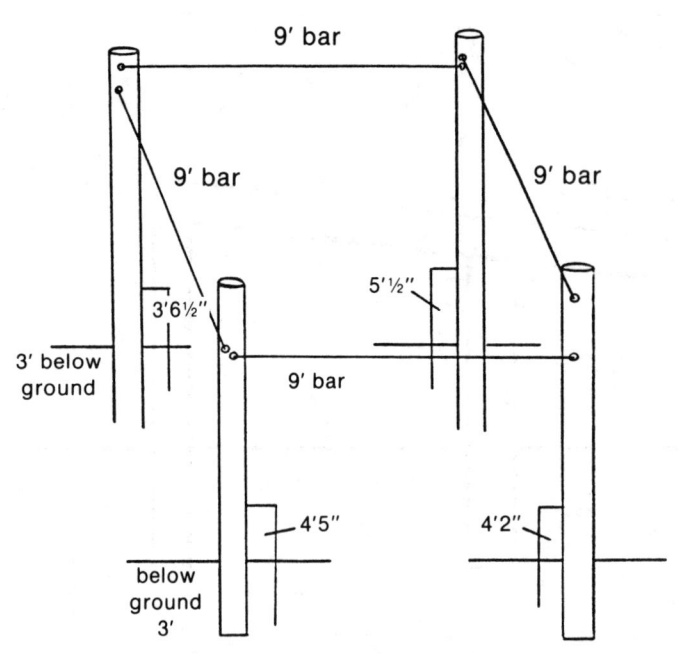

lowest bar is 5 feet off the ground, the second — 6 feet, the third — 7 feet and the fourth bar — 8 feet off the ground.

LOG HOP

Wood:
2 X 12' logs — 5" diameter

Hardware & Supplies:
3 bolts
3 washers

Holes:
1

Signs:
1 exercise sign
1 arrow

Construction Details:

12' — 5" diameter

(A heavy log is set permanently in the ground so it won't move.)

SHUTTLE RUN

Wood:
3 X 12' logs — 5" diameter

Hardware & Supplies:
3 bolts
3 washers

Holes:
3

Signs:
1 exercise trail
1 arrow

Construction Details:

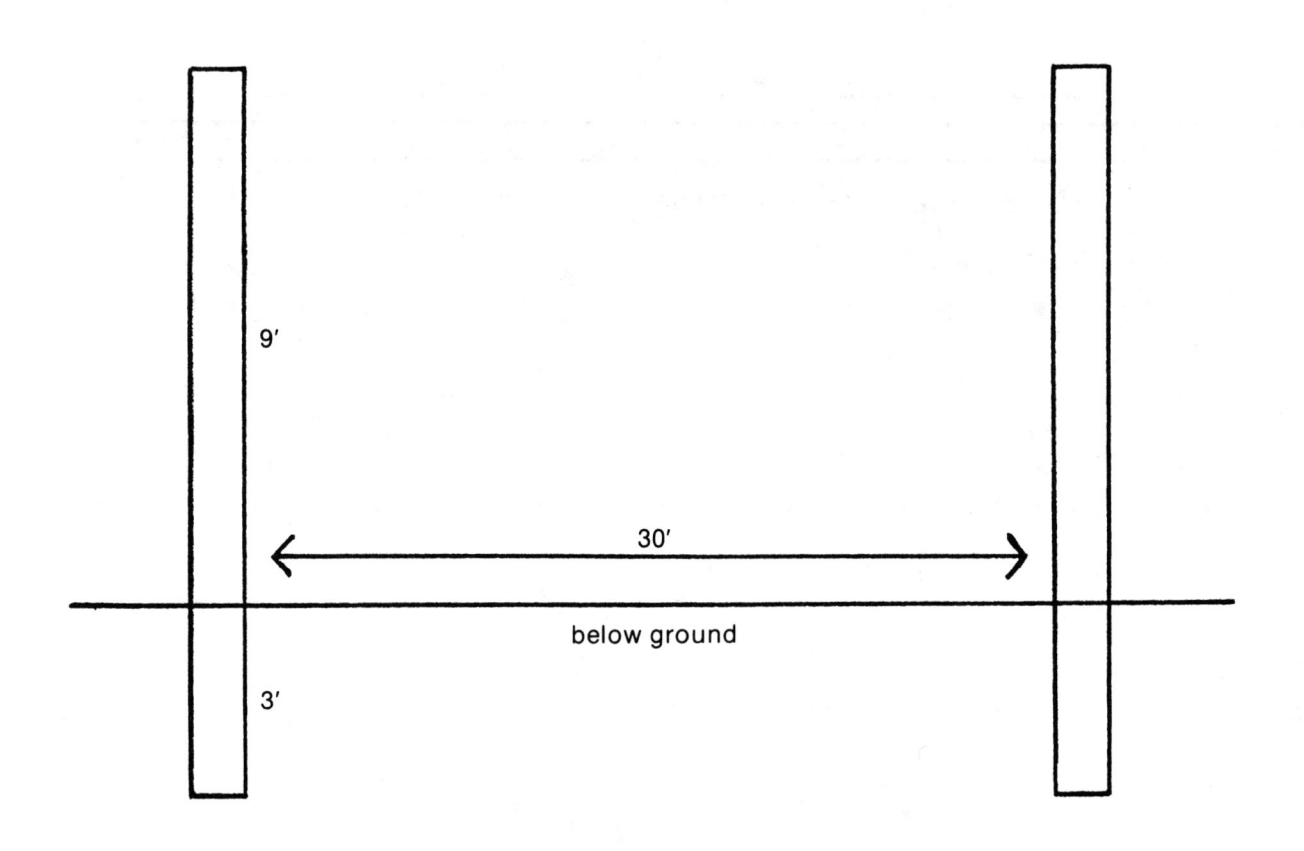

9'

30'

below ground

3'

INCLINED ARM PUSHUPS

Wood:
1 X 12' log — 5" diameter
1 X 7' log — 5" diameter
1 X 10'8" log — 5" diameter
1 X 5'7" log — 5" diameter

Hardware & Supplies:
3 bolts
3 washers
2 spikes — 10" long

Holes:
3

Signs:
1 exercise sign
1 arrow

Construction Details:

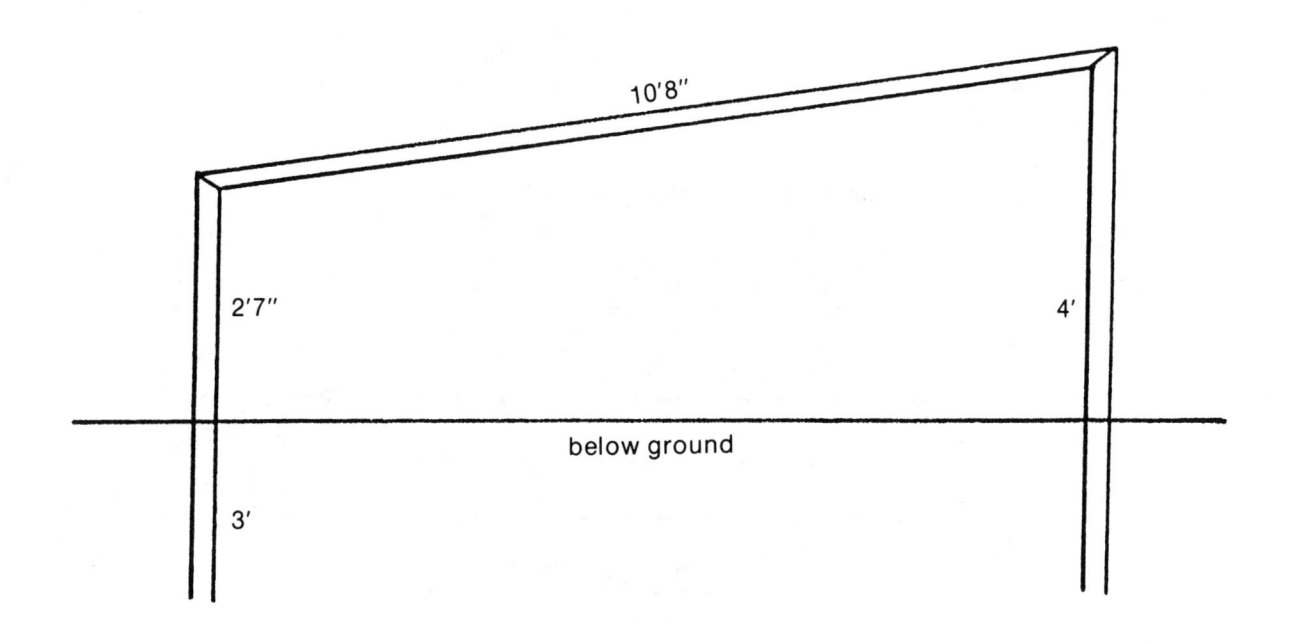

BALANCE BEAM

Wood:
1 X 12' log — 5" diameter
6 railway ties—8' long, 5½" X 7½" creosoted

Hardware & Supplies:
5 bolts
5 washers
9 spikes — 10" long

Holes:
1

Signs:
1 exercise sign
1 finish sign
1 arrow

Construction Details:

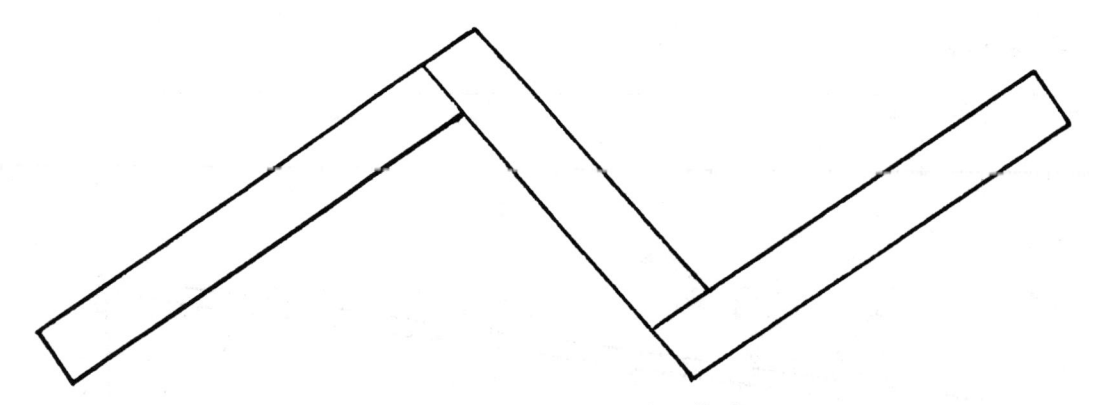

6 railway ties — 3 on bottom, 3 nailed on top.

spikes

(use 2 spikes per end)

Sample Publicity Pamphlet

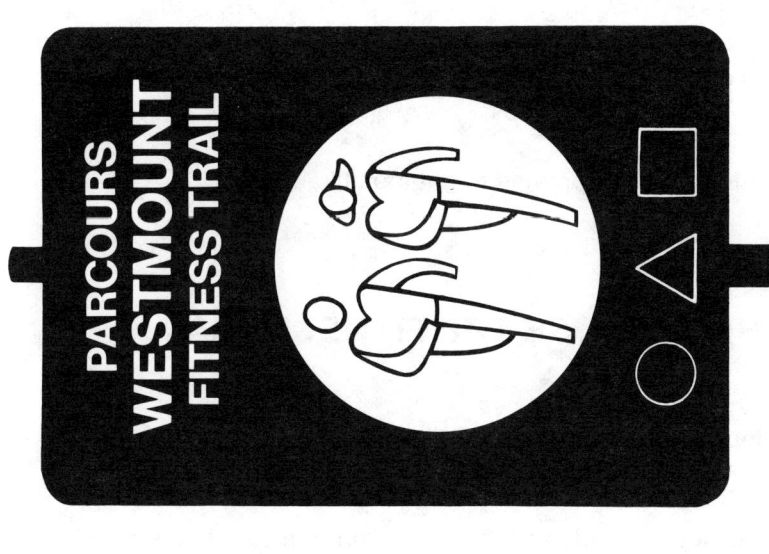

WESTMOUNT FITNESS TRAIL

The idea of the Fitness Trail is a European one which began in Switzerland during the last decade. The first trail was built by the Vita Life Insurance Company through a section of woods near Zurich in the interest of encouraging the Swiss to exercise while enjoying the woodland scenery.

The main attraction of the Fitness Trail is that it makes what to some is unpleasant calisthenics, seem more appealing through the addition of scenic woodlands and fresh air.

The Westmount Jogging Trail is the second of its kind in Quebec. The jogging circuit is 7/10 of a mile and contains 9 exercise stations. At the start, a bilingual sign shows how to use the trail. Each station has a plaque instructing the participant to perform a specific exercise a suggested number of times. At some of the exercise stations appropriate equipment such as chin up bars, are installed. These are adaptable to all ages, heights and sexes.

The exercise stations are designed in a careful progression with warm up exercises first, more strenuous exercises from stations 1 through 6 ending with warm down exercise for the remaining stations.

The Fitness Trail is not designed as a muscle building program, but rather as a cardiovascular (heart-lung-circulatory system) training circuit for various age groups. For best results, participants should work out 3 or 4 times a week gradually working up to the advanced level suggested number of exercise repetitions. Participants would be advised to try to improve their individual time rather than competing against other participants. Keeping a Fitness Trail Diary to record all performance data, pulse rate and weight after each session enables the users to keep a record of fitness progress.

All participants would be advised to have a complete medical before using the trail.

So come on out! It's free, open 24 hours a day, 7 days a week and it's outdoors.

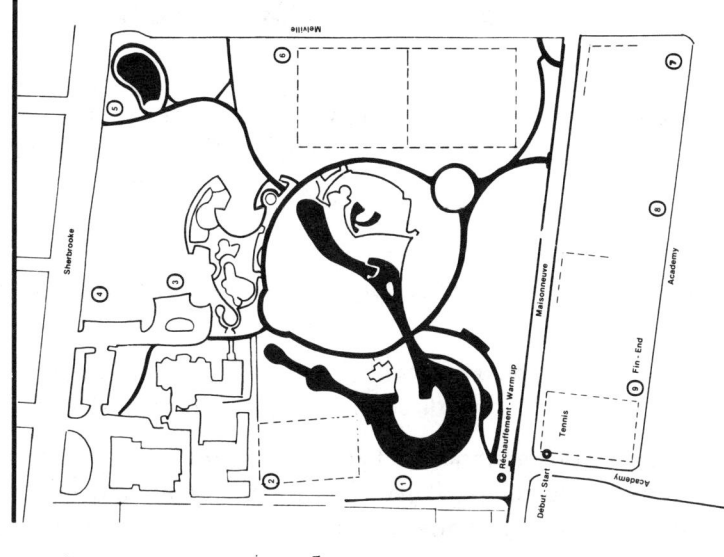

Figure 23

FITNESS TRAIL PROMOTION

Good publicity is an essential part of the promotion of your fitness trail. Flyers, posters, articles in newspapers, and periodic ads on radio and television will draw the public's attention to your trail.

Here are other steps you can take to encourage its use:

1. Plan an opening ceremony which involves local dignitaries, covered by the press, radio, and television.

2. Provide supervision the first few weeks the trail opens to assist participants; answer questions on how to properly use the fitness trail; give directions on parking, location of washrooms, etc.

3. Maintenance is a key factor in promoting use of your fitness trail. Frequent checks must be made to repair equipment and signs. Wood chips, if used, should be replaced when necessary. Washrooms must be kept clean, and removal of garbage and litter will also keep the fitness trail area attractive.

4. Prepare a short brochure containing general information on your fitness trail. A sample brochure might look like the one in Figure 23.

5. Distribute this brochure to local schools, fitness groups, recreation departments, diet organizations, local boys' and girls' clubs (e.g., Boy Scouts, Girl Guides, 4-H clubs) with a cover letter announcing the opening of your fitness trail and the conditions under which these groups may use it, receive additional information, etc.

6. If a second language is common among the people who are potential users of your fitness trail, make your short brochure and other publicity bilingual.

7. A detailed brochure may be necessary, particularly when your fitness trail first opens. It should give exact details on such topics as how to use the trail, where to start, facilities available, how to do the exercises and use the equipment provided, use of the trail in the winter, the short circuit, the importance of warming up and cooling down, how to follow a pulse rate-based exercise program such as the fitness trail.

This brochure provides invaluable information to participants, particularly when the fitness trail is first opened and people are becoming accustomed to the concept. A pamphlet box at the start of your fitness trail would hold these brochures.

A sample of the type of information to provide might look like this:

HOW TO USE THE FITNESS TRAIL

"At the start you will find a large sign which will tell you how to use the course. A map will show you where you will be going. Follow the numbered signs to all stations along the trail.

On your first trip through, proceed slowly so that you understand each exercise thoroughly. At each station you will find a plaque which will tell you how many repetitions to do of that particular exercise.

The number in the circle ⑤ tells the beginner how many repetitions to do; in this case 5. The triangle △10 indicates the repetitions for a person of intermediate level fitness, e.g., 10; and the square [15] shows the advanced people how many repetitions to do, e.g., 15.

If you don't know at which level to start, commence at the beginner's level. Every time you come to an exercise station, do the number of repetitions indicated in the circle. At a later date when you find these easy to accomplish, proceed to the intermediate level and so on to the advanced level.

You should expect to spend at least 6 weeks to 2 months at any given fitness level before you change to the next one. This is how long it takes the body to adapt to that particular level of exercise. Remember, for these exercises to be any good to you, you should exercise at least 3 to 4 times a week. Once a week will only hurt you unless you combine your use of the fitness trail with additional exercises during the week.

Start slowly and don't overdo it. Don't start your fitness program at the advanced level of repetitions. But remember that this is a cardiovascular training circuit so the idea is to run, jog, walk, or any combination of these between exercise stations."

FOLLOW UP

After the opening ceremony for your fitness trail, to ensure its continued use send the general pamphlet you wrote to local groups that might be interested in making use of the trail. Include local schools, health clubs, YMCAs, city recreation departments, diet organizations, and boys' and girls' organizations such as Boy and Girl Scouts, for instance.

Provide information on where the fitness trail is located, when it may be used, the name of a contact person to answer any inquiries, and details on how to use it.

Special events held at the fitness trail may also draw attention to its existence. Periodic coverage in newspapers and on radio and television will also help publicize the trail.

MAINTENANCE

To enhance the overall look of the fitness trail and to ensure the physical safety of participants, regular maintenance is essential.

Immediate repair of damaged equipment is vital to ensure that no accidents occur. Clean surroundings and well-kept grounds will make use of the fitness trail a pleasant experience. Thus garbage must be picked up regularly, and washrooms and associated facilities must be well maintained. A clean environment will also encourage users to take care of the trail.

Periodically, signs may need to be repainted or replaced as well. Seasonal maintenance may also be required with changes in weather.

BIBLIOGRAPHY

British Columbia Ministry of Health, *PAR-Q Validation Report,* May 1978.

Cooper, Kenneth H., *The Aerobics Way,* Bantam, New York, 1977, p. 52.

You and Your Heart Rate, Fitness and Amateur Sport, Government of Canada, Ottawa, 1978.

Morehouse, Laurence E., and Leonard Gross, *Total Fitness in 30 Minutes a Week,* Simon and Schuster, New York, 1975, p. 131.

Stamler et al, *Peoples Gas Company Study,* in *You and Your Heart Rate,* Fitness and Amateur Sport, Government of Canada, Ottawa, 1978.

"Woes of the Weekend Jock," *Time,* August 21, 1978, p. 50.

JUDY GILL, Ph.D

Judy Gill is a 36 year old Canadian, born in Ontario and raised in Quebec. A graduate of Macdonald College (1968), she obtained her Bachelor of Physical Education from McGill University (1970), a Masters in Physical Education from the University of Ottawa (1974), and a Ph.D. from the University of Oregon (1979).

Dr. Gill's knowledge of sports is exceptional. As a player, she participated and excelled in six athletic sports during high school, college and the university level. For over 12 years she has taught, coached and coordinated team and individual activities in more than 25 sports and fitness areas at the high school, college and adult educations levels.

Her many accomplishments include being the past secretary of the Quebec Olympic Wrestling Federation, a founding member of Outward Bound in Quebec (an organization dedicated to survival in the outdoors), a course director several times for the National Lifeguard and Red Cross Instructors Courses (both the highest awards in Canada in their respective areas), a founding member of Women's Ice Hockey in Quebec, (a representative to the Quebec University Athletic Association), and Athletic Director for Women for both Macdonald and John Abbott Colleges simultaneously.

The combination of her Masters and Doctoral degrees in physical education and administration has kept Dr. Gill in demand as a speaker and consultant in the fields of fitness, computers, motivational seminars and business--including organizations such as Coca-Cola, Rhone-Poulenc Pharma Inc., and the National Intramural-Recreational Sports Association, to name a few.

Because of her expertise, she also teaches subjects such as administration, theory of physical fitness, and computer applications in physical education and recreation. As Coordinator of Physical Fitness Testing at John Abbott College, she computerized this service to be compatible both with a main frame computer and an IBM PC.

A recognized fitness expert, Dr. Gill has studied fitness trails in Europe and North America. She has planned and helped build numerous trails including the unique Macdonald-Abbott and the Westmount Fitness Trails which are open 24 hours a day all year long.

Dr. Gill has acted as a co-host of Canadian radio programs as well as presenting fitness tips on both radio and television.

A GUIDE TO BUILDING FITNESS TRAILS is Judy Gill's sixth book, having written five previous books on the subjects of fitness, nutrition and games. She also writes a regular column for "Homemaker's Magazine," and has written numerous articles for magazines and periodicals.

St. Scholastica Library
Duluth, Minnesota 55811
WITHDRAWN